Me, Bea, CANCER Free

LIFE BEYOND A
BREAST CANCER
DIAGNOSIS

Me, Bea, CANCER Free

A KINDLY **BLUNT** *reflection on life, hope and thriving after cancer.*

HELEN BULLEN

Me, Bea, Cancer Free:

A KINDLY BLUNT reflection on reclaiming life, hope, and thriving after cancer.

Copyright © 2025 by Helen Bullen Publishing.

Kindly Blunt is a trademark of Helen Bullen.

All rights reserved. No part of this book may be reproduced or transmitted in any form or by any means, electronic or mechanical, including photocopying, recording or by any information storage and retrieval system without written permission of the publisher, except for the inclusion of brief quotations in a review.

ISBN 978-1-7392569-7-5 (Trade Paperback)
ISBN 978-1-7392569-8-2 (eBook)
ISBN 978-1-7392569-9-9 (Audiobook)

Editing by Melanie Scott - https://reedsy.com/melanie-scott

Proofreading by Eddie Sinden (my long suffering husband)

Cover Design – https://100covers.com

Interior Design by Helen Bullen – https://helenbullen.com

Cover photo by Andy Newbold https://www.newboldphotography.com/

Section Image credit to Convit; Shutterstock Image: 47636323

For my husband Eddie

Thank you for standing by me in the dark and helping me find the light again.

PROLOGUE

I chose to write a second book once I experienced the next part of my story of being "cancer free". This should be an exciting time filled with happiness and relief, and for a short while it really was. Then the reality of cancer returning and those around me expecting me to bounce back like nothing had happened started to kick in. I wrote this book for a few reasons. First, I used it as my own form of therapy. I wrote down my thoughts and observations as I struggled through this unexpectedly difficult phase of the journey. Writing acted as a medium to help my emotions and I always felt some relief from the anxiety when I wrote things down. Of course, I will be forever grateful to be one of the fortunate ones who gets a second chance, but this gratitude soon led to guilt at being a survivor when others didn't get the same opportunity. Writing it didn't make me feel any less lost and quite frankly terrified of cancer returning. I knew that this was a story I should share to help others going through it, to inform loved ones who support a survivor and as always to help people who are unsure what to say and how to act around someone who has been on this crap journey. I want this book to be a reminder to everyone to check their body. Take notice of how your body feels, and if you have any symptoms that are not usual for you, please go to see your GP for their expert opinion. Don't wait to get expert advice. Don't worry about being an inconvenience or that you are making a fuss. If you feel something is not your normal, get yourself seen ASAP.

As you read, you will see Kindly Blunt boxes sprinkled throughout, offering extra insights in my usual direct, no-nonsense style. I've always been straight-talking, with no time for sugar-coating. Instead I like to give practical advice to get things done. I run a business membership and one day one of my members summed up my approach as "kindly blunt". It was perfect and it stuck, because that's exactly what I am. I am kind and empathetic, but never one to tiptoe around the truth. I loved the term Kindly Blunt so much that I trademarked it, used it as the title for my podcast and it now appears in all of my books.

I want to share my story, help others and learn from my own words to help me move forward. Thank you for being part of my therapy; I hope you find the book informative and spot the snippets of my humour in parts.

Let me start as I mean to go on with your first Kindly Blunt box.

> **KINDLY BLUNT ADVICE**
>
> I want this book to also be a reminder to you to check your body. This book is about breast cancer so it seems right to remind you to do a self-check before you read anymore of this book. Although women are most at risk of breast cancer it does occur in men too, so please, whoever you are, check now before you carry on reading.

Contents

INTRODUCTION	1
Who The Hell Are Agnes And Bea?	
LIFE WITHOUT AGNES	4
Me, Bea, Cancer Free	
Taking Off Without Agnes	
Tears Of Absolute Relief	
Hit A Girl When She Is Down	
THIS IS NOT OVER	12
Brush Myself Off And Bounce Back	
The House Does Not Have A Door	
Life-Saving Mammogram	
I Am Far From Fine	
Guilt Of Being Well	
TOM THUMB	20
Unexpected Symptoms	
I'm A Hot Mess	
A DARK SHADOW LURKING	26
Cancer Free	
Anxiety	
TO CUT A LONG STORY SHORT	32
Happy Diagnosis Day	
The Guilt Is Strong	

A YEAR ON 36
    I Feel Like No One Cares
    Let Me See Another Christmas
    What A Difference A Year Makes
    Alive Happy And Hopeful

PLASTIC SURGEON 41
    99 Percent Sure
    Plenty!
    Poor Bea
    Thank You For Being My Therapist
    Let Loose To Sail Alone

SHOW AND TELL 51
    Brave Women
    Engaged

LOSING MY SENSE OF REALITY 56
    I Am Not Frightened Of Death
    A Bubbles Sort Of Day

TRIGGERS 61
    Think Before You Speak
    My Words Were Triggering Too

LIFE-SAVING BINGO 66
    Two Stars
    House

JUST CHECKING 70
    Obsessed
    Concern And Black Shadows

BOOK LAUNCH 76
    Agnes, Bea, Cancer And Me Is Live
    Rejected

TALKING ABOUT MY BOOBS	79
I Have Funny Bones	
ONLY FOOLS AND HORSES	81
Peckham	
HAIR	83
I Lost My Personality	
A Wedding Celebration	
Great Shoes	
Fingers Up To Cancer Today	
A DILEMMA	94
I Miss My Clea	
My World Is Turned Upside Down	
Polo-Neck Knickers	
BUILD A BOOB	99
Sewing Bea	
Meat In The Butcher Shop	
Oh Poop	
I Have Made A Mistake	
Fingers Crossed	
A Real Boob	
FABULOUS HOLIDAY	112
In A Pickle	
Rum!	
Bubbling Under The Surface	
DEM BONES	118
Infusions	
FREEDOM	122
Escape	

YEARLY CHECK — 124
    Poor Bea
    Smoke Coming Out Of My Ears

LOU'S HEN — 127
    Hens And Cakes

BARBIE BODY — 129
    Embrace Every Wrinkle
    My Precious Life
    Tattoo

MOTHER OF THE BRIDE — 135
    Exactly Three Years
    The Wedding

LEAVE A REVIEW — 140

GRATITUDE — 141

ABOUT THE AUTHOR — 143

JOIN MY COMMUNITY — 145

INTRODUCTION

Who The Hell Are Agnes And Bea?

My first book was called *Agnes, Bea, Cancer and Me* You may have read it but if by chance you have picked up this book as your first read of my story then I need to explain some things. Agnes was part of my life for 54 years but she had to go. Bea is still with me and you will have seen her mentioned already in the title of this book.

I was diagnosed with Stage 3 triple negative breast cancer in my right breast in July 2021. I wrote *Agnes, Bea, Cancer and Me* as a diary of my time from first diagnosis to getting the all clear, a long and gruelling nine months later. I realised early on in the book that I didn't quite know what to call my boobs. Here is what I wrote at the very start of my journey in that book:

"Do I call it a breast or a boob, as neither seems right? I need to give my breasts/boobs names. They have become a very personal yet public part of my body right now. I decided to call my right breast Agnes and the left Bea. A & B for short. I suppose I should tell you why I had a favourite side. Agnes has always been my favourite. She had a better shape. Agnes has always stood proud quite literally, and generally, I liked her best; she looked better than Bea. How bad do I now feel for Bea, who I had looked at as a second-class body part all my life. Agnes has got herself into trouble. A whole lot of trouble. Just like a poor maths student, Agnes's cell division is wrong. She can't

divide, add up, or multiply without making cellular-level mistakes. Her cell division is shit! She has been left to her own devices without correction, and now the damage is done. It seems she had decided to share her mathematical errors with my lymph nodes too. She has to be stopped, and fast. I don't love Agnes anymore. I ignore her and wear a bra night and day so that I just don't have to see her. I am in denial that Agnes has cancer. Instead, I am fixated on being mad at her mathematic capabilities, or should I say lack of them."

Moving on nine months and a whole book later, I can say proudly, I quite literally got Agnes off my chest. A right-sided mastectomy and I am left with Bea, my one and only, on the left side of my chest. I miss Agnes, but I am unlikely to tell you that out loud. I have not forgotten her lack of mathematical ability in her division of cells. I have not forgiven her for getting things wrong and passing that incorrect information onto my lymph nodes too. I do, however, miss the normality of her being around. Boobs normally come in pairs and now Bea is alone. Bea needed Agnes to make up a full cleavage. Bea misses her to nestle up to. Agnes was the "clea" to Bea's "vage". Bea is left in a world of asymmetry but I am thankful she is still with me and healthy. This book is about my journey post cancer. Some may assume it is simple and without any troubles or cares but the reality is very different and I shall be sharing my thoughts on the way.

Bea
My One
And Only

LIFE WITHOUT AGNES

"I have huge guilt that I am a survivor"

Me, Bea, Cancer Free

I finished my last book *Agnes, Bea, Cancer and Me* on my honeymoon. Agnes was gone, I was cancer free and ready to live life. It seems appropriate to restart my story there, but first a small recap to set the scene.

Eddie, my husband, and I had the initial date for our wedding planned for 9th May 2020. We had been together for over 15 years and decided in 2020 we would get married, but as you well know 2020 was the year the world went into lockdown. Our initial wedding date was postponed. With a small window of restrictions being lifted, we managed to get married with just six other people on 18th July 2020. Our children, my parents and one friend who is also a registrar turned up at the local registry office and the official ceremony was done. As we knew we would dress up and party properly when the world reopened, Eddie and I turned up in our jeans and trainers and celebrated, at a distance, with a handful of friends in our garden, with takeaway pizza and tubs of Ben & Jerry's. It was pretty perfect.

The first Big C, Covid, stopped our first planned celebrations in 2020 and then the year after, the second Big C, Cancer, stopped those celebrations once again as I underwent six months of intense chemotherapy. Finally, in May 2022, I walked down the aisle with just 1cm of hair, one boob and a few extra stones of weight. It was a fabulous day despite my appearance - not the way I planned but I was alive, cancer free and I had married my best friend, Eddie.

Taking Off Without Agnes

After all we had gone through, we decided our honeymoon was going to be special and to be honest I had no confidence that I would survive long enough to see any more holidays after this one. Despite being given the "no sign of cancer" and everyone around me believing I would feel instant relief, I feel very different. Every day still feels like a bonus and I feel there is no time to waste waiting to do things. However, my expectations of cancer staying away are low and I am determined, no matter how long I have left, I will continue to move forward smiling as much as I can.

We had booked three weeks in the Seychelles and during that time we will be staying in quality hotels with private pools, villas over the water, travelling to three of the islands. We set off to the airport a few days after our delayed wedding celebrations. I honestly feel like I am running away from the reality of cancer, chemotherapy, operations and hospitals. This journey is not over, but I am going to escape for three full weeks and do my very best to forget it happened.

Today is the first time through an airport without Agnes. I will be taking off without her, but today I have a new worry: my false boob. First, let me tell you a bit about false boobs. I was kindly given a prosthetic boob from the NHS and I am honestly grateful.

I remember going to be fitted for this type of boob; it was an interesting visit. It was just like going to a shoe shop with a cupboard full of cardboard boxes with different styles and sizes. Styles such as "perky", "almost perky" and in my case "serious droop". Of course they are not labelled that way, but they may as well have been. Poor old Bea has a natural droop, so the false boob had to be matched to her. I remember the nurse looking at Bea and assessing how to match her. "Ahh," she said with a happy nod, "we will need one with a bigger natural droop, try this one". If you have read my books before, you know I have a sense of humour and this was no different. I couldn't help but let out a huge laugh. Talk about unintentionally knocking a girl when she is down. I drove home with my new "droopy" size 8 silicone boob sat on the passenger seat beside me. That's when it dawned on me that my boob size matches my UK trainer size. I wonder if we all have feet the same size as our boobs? Did you just look down at your feet to check?

Looky-Likey boob, as it shall now forever be known, actually looks like a boob. It is the same colour as my skin, with a bump where a real nipple would be. Being so lifelike is not that useful when a person like me is prone to whipping it out and slapping it on the table when it gets uncomfortable. To touch it feels like touching a stress ball. I do wonder why it needs to look so real as all I need is a boob shape to go under my clothes. Instead I have a slightly obscene, stress boob. A whole new take on items you can have on your office desk to reduce stress.

Looky-Likey also needs a special bra to sit in. The bras I bought to house her are best described as functional. Not long after my mastectomy, I bought three bras that were all the same style in different colours: white, neutral and black. I like the black one best as it has a little bit of lace covering the seriously structured bra. In the white bra, my chest takes on a pointed silhouette and it gives me a similar look to that of Madonna in her infamous pink cone bra outfit created for her by Gaultier. I try singing when I wear this bra, but I have not noticed any pop star tendencies yet. The neutral-coloured bra is just horrid. In my opinion, no one should buy a neutral-coloured bra if they want in anyway to feel pretty. I understand it's a functional shade but this bra's shape and colour makes me feel really frumpy. Never buy matching neutral bra and knickers because if you do we can never be friends.

Back to my story about my new worry. I am at the airport with Looky-Likey nestled into the pocket section of the scaffolding of my bra. I am about to go through airport security with a prosthetic boob and I have read somewhere that there was a possibility that it could react to the plane's air pressure. I have visions of it swelling up on the flight and, worse, exploding as we soar high into the sky. I can imagine the media frenzy reporting a story about a woman travelling to the Seychelles when one of her boobs enlarged to the size of a Swiss ball just before exploding. Further reports would refer to this as a major security alert, with the female being restrained as the flight was rerouted for an emergency landing.

Of course, that was never going to happen, but when I read the guidance on Looky-Likey's box it explains that air pressure on a flight can cause air bubbles to form inside. My worry, however, is more imminent as I am about to go through security. I am in the queue wondering how I will explain things if I am pulled aside. Will I freak out security, set off alarms, or even be accused of having a boob stuffed with drugs? This is, of course, a complete overreaction but right now it is a very real worry for me. I am not yet used to having just Bea on my chest. I regularly outwardly tell others that I don't care that I have lost Agnes, but the truth is, I do care. My life has been turned upside down with so many new things I have had to get used to, from self-injections, blood tests, chemotherapy and mastectomy as just a few examples. Change is hard for anyone, but when you go through a cancer journey the changes are daily and extreme. I am in a state of shock despite outwardly looking like I have it all together.

I sail through security and of course no one is bothered except for me. I am not the only person that will pass through security with a false boob and they must be very used to it. Just before we board our flight, I decide to take the Looky-Likey out of my bra and put it in my hand luggage. Although it's a ridiculous worry, I don't want to be the lady on the plane whose boob explodes, and I will deny all knowledge if it does.

Being given the "no sign of cancer" is a luxury not everyone is given and I am truly grateful that my story followed this path. However, I have huge guilt that I am a survivor when others were not given that chance. I thought getting through all the treatment to rid me of the cancer was going to be a time to celebrate, but that only lasted a few days. Friends and family celebrated but automatically expected me be the person I was before all of this. Post-treatment, I find I worry about almost everything in my life. I am desperate to find the "old me" that existed before cancer rocked my world. Instead I find a new version and I don't like what I have become.

KINDLY BLUNT MESSAGE

If you are post-treatment and feel like a stranger to your old self, please know you are not alone. Treatment leaves scars both physical and emotional, and healing takes time. There is no "right" way to feel after going through something so life-altering. Be patient with yourself. Let the tears flow when they need to, smile whenever you can and, most importantly, give yourself the grace to recover fully, at your own pace. P.S. Of course prosthetic boobs won't explode during a flight – sorry if I worried you.

Tears Of Absolute Relief

When you go through the journey of cancer treatment, it feels like you are on a conveyor belt of tests, examinations, worry, anxiety, sadness and feeling the worst you have ever felt. I certainly felt this way. Although there were plenty of tears on my journey, I also realise that I went into survival mode. A head down, get on with it type of mentality. It's how I approach most things. Moments of melt-down, then a word with myself to pick myself up and put on a brave face so others don't know how I am feeling. During the treatments, it was my way of getting through the horror of chemotherapy and the abuse of my body to get a positive outcome. This, however, has taken its toll.

When you hold in real emotions for such a long time, they are likely to bubble to the surface when you least expect it. Here I am sitting on a plane, next to my husband, best friend and biggest supporter, flying to one of the most beautiful places on earth. Three weeks away in the Seychelles, island-hopping. I should be so happy, but as we take off, I lay my head on Eddie's shoulder and like a tsunami I break down in tears. Tears of absolute relief. Tears from months of trauma. An unstoppable stream of tears fall silently down my face. I didn't know at the time, but this type of crying was to be a common occurrence for many months to come.

The Seychelles is fabulous. My husband Eddie, who has also had cancer and chemotherapy treatment, fully understands the need to live our lives. He has gone all out on our stunning honeymoon accommodation and I am so grateful we are able to have this opportunity. We stay on three different islands and each time in beautiful surroundings with beach villas, private pools and mouth-watering food.

My favourite villa of our stay, is over the ocean, with a bathroom that has full-length glass doors looking over the water. I have not been able to have baths for months, due to the PICC line inserted into my arm whilst having chemo drugs and then a mastectomy scar that was not allowed to get wet. Now, every day, I run a full bath and relax into the bubbles looking out at the incredible view. A stunning memory made. Making memories is so important to me. Memories of a life well lived, no matter how long I have left.

Hit A Girl When She Is Down

This is the first time I have been away with only Bea. A long scar is all that remains where Agnes once sat. I don't mind my scar now the stitches are gone and the redness has subsided. I see it as my battle scar. If you look carefully at my first book *Agnes, Bea, Cancer and Me*, you will notice that the cover photo is me proudly standing tall with my scar visible. I feel like a warrior and I have the scars to prove it.

Nothing is normal when you finish treatment, and just having Bea is a big adjustment. I don't have much hair yet either and I miss it. Yes, it is starting to grow back and of course the one chin hair I used to have before treatment has grown back with full force. I am impatient to get my old look and life back and I don't want to wait any longer. I lost my hair in August 2021 and it's now May 2022, and although I am grateful it is starting to come back, it is still very short. I am two stone heavier from the steroids and lack of exercise. I am far from my old self.

The last stop of our holiday is a return back to the mainland of Mahe, where we will catch our flight home. As we go through passport control, I am pulled aside by a serious-looking border guard and asked why I don't look like my passport. He tells me he is not sure I am the same person. Talk about hit a girl when she is down. The passport scanning machine does not recognise my face and now the customs man is stern and a little frightening. Perhaps I have watched too many episodes of *Border Security* on TV, as I imagine I shall be interrogated as a suspect drug mule. Instead, I tell the man the truth that I have been through cancer treatment. In an instant, the very intimidating and stern man is showing concern, wishing me well and ushering me through his zone. An odd moment and a realisation that I have a long way to go before I look like I used to. I worry I may never get that person back and I feel incredibly sad.

THIS IS NOT OVER

"Bleached blonde hair and a fake boob"

Brush Myself Off And Bounce Back

It would be easy, looking in from the outside, to think that my cancer journey is done and my life is back to normal. Everyone thinks it's all finished and now only a few people check in on me. The reality is my world is still full of check-ups, blood tests, examinations and possibly reconstruction surgery. My world is also full of constant worry. I try not to talk about cancer, but it is always there in the back of my mind. I want to talk about it, but people are reluctant to listen. It is like a form of PTSD that people don't understand. Of course, people understand it is hard when you go through cancer, but afterwards I am expected to brush myself off and bounce back and forget it all. In reality the scars are deep, both mentally and physically. There is a constant worry that won't leave me alone and tears flow in private over the smallest of things. Fear of ill-health is heightened, and no longer can I think, "that will never happen to me". I am not unhappy, just in extreme shock over what I have been through. I had no time when I was diagnosed to process the reality of the situation, I just had to get on with it. Now the dust has settled, everyone assumes I have moved on without a care in the world. A chapter in my life that has passed. Instead, I have moved onto the next chapter, which is different but equally scary. What makes it hard is that I am expected to hold it all inside me. I wasn't sure if this book would be written when I finished "*Agnes, Bea, Cancer and Me*" but I soon realised that being post-cancer has its own set of problems and I want to put my story out there to share how it feels after cancer treatment is over. I hope it helps others realise they are not alone and raises awareness to onlookers that the journey continues despite it appearing like it is all over.

The House Does Not Have A Door

I was diagnosed with triple negative (TN) breast cancer and I think it is important to explain more about this type of breast cancer, as my treatment after the "all clear" is different from many other types. Triple negative breast cancer is not hormone related. The cells do not have receptors for oestrogen, progesterone and human epidermal growth factor receptor 2 (HER2), hence the name triple negative. It accounts for just 15 percent of all breast cancers. Many women with TN breast cancer have a mutation in their BRCA 1 and BRCA 2 genes. This mutation means cells have the ability to grow out of control. I had genetic testing done early on in my diagnosis and I was very fortunate to find that I don't have the BRCA gene mutation. However the genetics team will keep my sample on file should they discover another gene that has predisposed me to this type of cancer that may not have been discovered yet. Not having any BRCA gene mutation is a relief for me and for my family. There is not much to be thankful for when you have cancer, but I am so thankful for that and I know this makes me incredibly lucky. I am acutely aware that not everyone is as lucky as me.

As TN breast cancer is not hormone related, the treatment for this type of breast cancer is limited. Someone once described the difference to me in very simple terms. They told me to imagine that breast cancer is a house. With hormone related breast cancer that house has a door and the medical team have a variety of keys they can use to unlock it (the keys being treatments to block hormones). However in TN cancer the house does not have a door, let alone any keys to get in. The usual treatment protocol for TN breast cancer is strong chemotherapy followed by mastectomy and then, for most, radiotherapy. It is more aggressive than most breast cancers and the recurrence rate is high.

I was fortunate that after 16 chemotherapy infusions, a unilateral mastectomy and complete axillary (armpit area) node clearance, testing of the surgically removed tissue, revealed no sign of cancer. The chemotherapy had destroyed all the cancer cells. I did not have to continue with further chemotherapy or radiotherapy. Again I consider myself very lucky. It was a tough journey but it could have been much worse. Post-treatment, hormone-related breast cancers are given an adjuvant treatment of hormone therapy to lower the chances of it returning. As TN is not hormone related, hormone therapy will not help prevent the return of this type of cancer. Instead I have to keep my fingers crossed and hope I can get to five years clear, as the odds of my survival increase at that point. TN breast cancer, if it returns, tends to come back quickly. I am currently on a 60:40 split, in my favour, for it not to return. I have my fingers crossed extra tight that I stay cancer free. Post-treatment, I am being given, over three years, a course of six-monthly zoledronic acid infusions to keep my bones strong. Zoledronic acid, a bisphosphonate, reduces the activity of the cells that break down bone cells, osteoclasts. It is hoped that this can reduce the risk of cancer spreading to the bones. It also helps to keep my bones strong now that I am post menopause.

Life-Saving Mammogram

It's exactly a year since I had the routine mammogram that saved my life. It is the June extended bank holiday for the Queen's Platinum Jubilee. Eddie is away in France with his mates, so I am home alone. I decide to visit my daughter, which is always a nice thing to do. I laugh as I drive to her house as I am conscious my false boob is rising as I go. It gets so high it almost hits my chin, so with one swift move I pull it out and dump it on the seat next to me. I am very happy to go without it as I just can't be arsed with it today. Better hope I don't get pulled over as it may take some explaining.

My daughter and I go out for a lovely walk followed by a coffee. It is amazing how the smallest of things are of great pleasure to me now. My daughter is celebrating moving to her new house exactly a year ago. I don't say anything but it dawns on me that her moving day was the same day I went for my mammogram a year ago. The day cancer was spotted and, although I did not know it on that day, it was the day that saved my life. It has been a hell of a year and I can't explain the relief I feel being alive a year on, enjoying time with my beautiful daughter. Things could have been very different and I am so grateful I made it to the other side of treatment. It is now June 2022 and I am starting to get back to many things that I did before the whole cancer nightmare. It feels good, although I have to admit my confidence has been knocked. Before cancer I was really confident but now I worry over the smallest things, with bouts of crippling anxiety. I am not sure if this is PTSD or symptoms of being pushed through menopause on fast track. I guess it is a bit of both. Today, I need to get my confidence mask on as I am off to a new business networking group. It is refreshing to be in an environment where no one knows I have had cancer. However, I feel conscious of my treatment past, as I rock up with an inch of bleached blonde hair and a fake boob tucked in my bra. Amusingly, it seems my appearance gives me a new persona and the first person I talk to assumes I am an artist. Another rushes over to chat as she says I "look interesting". Although I am desperate to get my old look back, today I quite like looking like a funky rock chick artistic type. It feels like a new start for me and I enjoy being known for my business acumen rather than for my cancer, although I have to admit to all that I am far from being a talented artist.

I Am Far From Fine

I don't want to be here. It's just a few months since I was given the "no sign of cancer" news. I have enjoyed a few months away from the multitude of hospital checks, examinations and treatments. The hospital was fantastic and it saved my life but, it is the last place in the world I want to be. June brings about new treatment and with that comes more blood tests and extra visits to the chemo ward. Although I no longer need chemotherapy, I have six infusions of zoledronic acid over the next three years. Today is my first infusion.

I have come on my own to the hospital, as Eddie is away. I put on a brave face and told him I would be fine on my own. Of course, that was a cover up as being here I am far from fine, but surely if I am cancer free I should be skipping down the ward full of the joys of spring. Unfortunately that is not how it feels, even if everyone else assumes it should be. Like it or not, I have to go back to the chemotherapy ward for this treatment. I start to panic as I really don't want to go near the chemotherapy wards ever again. Of course those wards and the angel nurses saved my life, but being back here brings back many terrible memories. I swear this must be what PTSD feels like. I struggle emotionally as I walk along the hospital corridors I have passed through so many times, on my way to the ward. This is a huge trigger and I am finding it hard to hold back the tears. I remember the staircase that I struggled to climb every week and the lift for when I just could not manage it. I find the clinical cleaning fluid smell that surrounds me an awful reminder of the past.

The same familiar reception staff sit behind the ward desk as I pass across my hospital card. I have had so many visits here that my first appointment card is full and I am half-way through the second one. I wait as the lady checks me in and allocates me a ward number to go to, I arrive at the ward and they ask me to go to a numbered chair. I am weighed, my blood pressure is taken and I can hear them preparing the bag of meds that I am about to have. The very same routine I had during chemotherapy: it doesn't feel good being back in this world. The only change is a few specific questions asked around my dental health. Although zoledronic acid is being administered to help my bone density, it can have serious side effects if not monitored carefully. The major concern is my teeth. Osteonecrosis can occur in the jaw, which means the bone in that area can die. How scary does that sound? I therefore have to be seen by a dentist on a regular basis and avoid any major dental work. Every time I arrive in the hospital they ask about my last dental visit as well as reviewing bloods taken a few days prior to the infusions. They test my kidneys and liver function and other things I have not yet worked out. Generally, I have to be in good health to take each infusion. Long-term use of the drug can cause fracture of the femur, which puzzles me as it goes against the theory that this drug will strengthen my bones. Apparently this risk is avoided by stopping the drug after a certain number of years. Last week I was instructed to get my teeth checked by my dentist before they would allow this infusion. I am not allowed to have any major work done on my teeth for the next four years so they are rightly concerned about my oral health. As a precaution, I have been given special toothpaste on prescription that has a higher concentration of fluoride to prevent cavities. This world post-cancer is not as easy as others assume.

All around me sick people are being given injections, transfusions, cold caps etc. Young, old, cancer does not discriminate, it's shit like that. Chemotherapy pumps are bleeping and I hate the triggering smell of the ward. A smell that brings back a flood of miserable memories. Today everyone in the ward with me looks really sick. I didn't notice how sick people looked when I was one of them, but today it really affects me. I hate this place, which seems wrong as it is an amazing place with such kind people working here, but the memories of going through treatment are like deep wounds that have been opened up as I sit here today. The memories of the chemotherapy are strong. I only told a few friends I am back to the ward today, as I feel I am not meant to mention cancer anymore. I have only told those people who asked how I am. I let everyone else think it is all over, as that seems to make them more comfortable. When I had cancer, people were uncomfortable around me and now I don't have cancer I feel I am expected to move on and spare any further worry for others. But here I am, holding back the tears still in a new world of anxiety.

Guilt Of Being Well

I feel so much guilt that I no longer have cancer. That may sound silly, but it is a real emotion for me. The guilt of being well when others are not so fortunate is huge. My hair is starting to grow back and I no longer struggle to walk to the hospital ward. I wish I had a T-shirt that told people I had been there, I had done my time and I understand what they are going through. I wish Eddie was here with me, but today I have to do this alone. I try to focus on getting through the infusion. The ward has new chairs and although they look smarter I find them uncomfortable. I don't have Percy the PICC line any more to make the infusion of drugs easy (a PICC line is a peripherally inserted central catheter, which in basic terms is a tube that is inserted into the upper arm so that drugs can be easily administered into the vein. It remains in place during the course of all your treatments). I am thankful I don't have a tube constantly in my arm anymore, but I hate having a cannula put into my hand for the zoledronic acid to be fed into my veins. Despite the care of the nurse, it hurts and it makes me feel sick seeing the needle. This infusion only takes about 20 minutes, far quicker than the hours I sat having chemotherapy drugs given. As the meds start to infuse into my system I focus hard on being grateful for being given another chance at life. I am out the door of the hospital in just over an hour and it's a huge relief to escape all the memories.

I have been told that I may feel like I have flu for a few days and that feels easy compared to recovering after chemotherapy. The next few days I feel a little under the weather but nothing severe. I ache a little and my joints hurt, but in the great scheme of things it is totally bearable. With Eddie being away, I rest longer in bed than usual over the next few days.

KINDLY BLUNT ADVICE

If you know someone who has gone through cancer, be aware that their journey will never be over. It will change and each person will have a different way of coping. Listen if someone wants to talk about it. Don't try and distract them or belittle their feelings. If they wish to remain silent about it all, then respect that too. Never tell them they should be "grateful they survived and to forget about it and move on". (Yes, that was said to me and no, it didn't help at all.)

TOM THUMB

"I have to get on with it"

Unexpected Symptoms

My mastectomy operation is a great success and, apart from some extreme pain when I was coming around immediately after the operation, it was relatively low-grade pain as I recovered. I do mourn the loss of Agnes, but she could not be trusted not to muck up her cell division again. The risk of cancer returning was too high to let her stay. Agnes is gone and with her went the cancer cells.

Despite the operation being a success, I do have other symptoms that I was not expecting to linger. Post-op, I have numbness in the back of my right arm. Light touch is hard to feel, but if I pinch myself it still hurts and yes, of course I have pinched myself a few times just to check. I have pins and needles in my right hand at the tips of all my fingers. I have my nails really short, as if they are longer typing is an effort and as a writer that is a problem. I was warned prior to the operation that there could be nerve damage. I am thankful that it is just sensory and not a reduced function of my muscles, which can happen in extreme cases. My surgeon did an amazing job and her stitching was extremely neat, and for that I am extremely grateful. I do think all surgeons should have a sample of their needlework hanging on their consultation room wall, like an embroidery sampler. I did suggest it to my surgeon in a moment of jest but she looked at me as if I was mad. Perhaps she has a point. My sense of humour can get me in trouble, but what do you think? Would it be a great idea for them to show their skills in cross-stitch for all to see? I think so.

My thumb has been a mystery for a while. I have a patch of dead skin in the centre of the pad of my right thumb. It looks as if I have burnt an area of my thumb pad, as the skin is shiny. If I press the shiny area, it stays indented and I have joked that it is from keeping Eddie under the thumb. Fortunately his forehead does not have a corresponding thumb impression or else I could be in real trouble. After taking some photos, it was agreed I needed to see a specialist skin doctor. Off I went with my thumb to show it to the expert. As is my way that thumb is now known as Tom. I see the specialist skin GP and she diagnoses Tom with skin damage post-chemotherapy. It had not even crossed my mind it was anything to do with my cancer treatment, but I do remember they warn you about peripheral neuropathy (nerve damage) in fingers and toes. I thought I was fortunate enough to have escaped this side effect, but it seems Tom was not so lucky. I have damage to a small area of my skin and in the great scheme of things it is a minor problem after the aggressive chemotherapy that saved my life. Eddie can tell people he is "under the thumb" and use the dent in Tom as evidence. Cancer really is the gift that keeps giving, but again I shall focus on being grateful for life. Not sure how Tom feels about it, however.

Since having chemotherapy I feel like I have aged 10 years. Prior to all of this I was fit and would regularly run 5-10 kilometres, with multiple sessions on the spin bike every week. Now I am left with a body that is two stone overweight and joints that feel like they need a good lubricant oil every morning. I am so stiff I have noticed I am struggling to get up off the floor. I am really worried, as I know it is not good for someone of my age to have such reduced range of movement. My retired osteopath brain kicks in, and I have set about learning how to move again. Every morning I come downstairs, put the coffee on and, while it is brewing, sit on the floor and practice getting myself back up. To begin with I have to shuffle to the kitchen units and pull myself up with them as my aid. I have been doing this three to five times every day and gradually my body has started to respond. Finally I can get back up without support. It is a relief that my body is responding and I have hope I may be able to turn things around. I have always been amazed how the body adapts to change in my work as an osteopath. I am however in disbelief that the person who used to train for marathons, me, is now reduced to training to get up off the floor, a simple skill I have always taken for granted. It is likely I will never know exactly what made my joints so stiff. Was it the chemotherapy, being pushed fast through menopause, or lack of exercise? It is likely it was a combination of them all. My consultant did suggest that the knee pain I now get is likely to have been from side effects of the chemotherapy. Another cancer gift I am not grateful for.

Weight gain is something that has upset me as much as losing my hair during treatment. Prior to all of this, I didn't think I was too hung up on my appearance, but it seems I am. I am not someone who needs a face of makeup and fancy clothes to step outside the door, but I do like to have nice hair and to look fit and athletic, or should I say I like to feel athletic at my age. Now I certainly don't feel athletic. Instead I feel ugly and heavy. None of my clothes fit and I am heavier than I was when I was pregnant with my children. Some people are surprised that someone who went through cancer treatment gained weight, but it's more common than you may think. Steroids, chemotherapy, lack of movement and, in my case, eating ice cream meant I packed on the weight. It feels really unfair after all the hard work I put into being strong prior to all of this. I have to remember to be thankful that I was strong before all the chemotherapy, as I do think it helped my body manage the poison. I am also forever grateful that I am alive.

All through this, I have been determined that cancer was not going to beat me despite the reality that I had no control over how it all turned out. I am now determined that cancer will not dictate how I look and feel. I may be determined, but returning to my old normal is going to be harder than I thought and secretly I know I will never be the same. Time to embrace a strong, confident new me. Time to eat well, keep exercising and live a full and wonderful life. If only it was as easy as typing that last sentence.

Yoga is my new, go-to, in my return to fitness and in my hope to regain my flexibility. I laugh every time I sit down to start a class as I find it almost impossible to cross my legs in any sort of yoga position and trying a child's pose is impossible when I can't fully flex my left knee anymore. I try to remind myself I have improved, as I can now get up and down off the floor. I have committed to doing yoga at least four times a week and gradually my body is relearning how to move more easily. I dread to think what I look like, but the lovely lady taking the online classes keeps saying not to worry and do what you can. "You are where you are meant to be" is a phrase that makes me giggle as I am trying to stick my bum up in the air whilst pushing my heels to the ground. A "downward dog" they call it. More like a "fat cow" in my case. Laughter is my medicine so "fat cow" is perfect, although it's hard to balance when giggling. The reality of yoga is I do struggle with some movements that involve my right breast scar. A mastectomy scar is restrictive, but with work my arm range of movement is returning and I am proud of the work I have done daily to get it back to normal. Being a retired osteopath, there is no way I am not going to do my rehab.

I'm A Hot Mess

I was almost 54 when I got my cancer diagnosis. I certainly had a few menopause symptoms starting, but they were vague symptoms that I would not have classed as problematic. Chemotherapy pushed me straight into menopause. Overnight I hit it head on, with full-on hot sweats, anxiety and stress. Not what you need when dealing with the side effects of chemotherapy, but what many women have to deal with during treatment. I am eternally grateful that I was not a younger woman who still wanted to have a family. I have my children and I have to remember it is just a natural process that I would be going through at my age, just not quite at the speed it happened. Going through chemotherapy was tough, but dealing with fast-track menopause didn't make it any easier.

Post-cancer, I still have severe menopause symptoms. Hot flushes, anxiety, brain fog, constantly needing a pee, especially at night, and the list of symptoms goes on. Hormone medication is not an option for me to help alleviate the symptoms. HRT (hormone replacement therapy) is not recommended after any type of breast cancer as my oncology team think the risk of recurrence is too high. Although Agnes has gone, they have explained that the risk to Bea getting cancer is increased and so HRT is not something they will support me having. I can't say I fully understand their reasoning, but it seems the answer is a firm "NO" from my team. I trust them and the "no" came from more than one expert, so I will respect that.

I have to get on with it, but that is easier said than done. I am of the age that most of my friends are on HRT and it seems that at every gathering people are talking about the benefits and how glad they are that they can get rid of the symptoms. Conversations explaining how they just could not put up with it and how the medication was much needed for their physical and mental health. Often this is said without any thought that I have no choice but to put up with it. What seems to make it worse right now is there is a positive promotion of HRT all over the media. Every daytime programme has experts talking about the benefits and it feels like they have forgotten the small minority of women who will never be able to take advantage of this type of medication. Instead, I am left to cope with a myriad of symptoms. This makes me feel down and angry that I can't access this so-called medical wonder drug. Of course, it is yet to be seen if the advice changes, but right now HRT is a hot topic, whilst I am left in a hot mess.

KINDLY BLUNT MOTIVATION

Don't be hard on your body after you have finished your cancer treatment. It will have changed and, although that can be upsetting, there are positives to focus on. Being alive is the first and then knowing that you can make changes. They may be slow but you can rebuild yourself. Embrace the new you and smile as often as you can. You are awesome.

A DARK SHADOW LURKING

"The scars are deep"

Cancer Free

I have a shadow and it is just behind me, lurking and ready to pounce. "Cancer free" does not feel that free. It feels like a dark shadow always behind me and I am desperately trying to stay a few steps ahead of it. Everyone else thinks you are done when you are told "no sign of cancer". In all the films patients are told "You are cancer free" and everyone celebrates. I imagined hearing the words "cancer free" then running to the oncologist, waiting with open arms to pick me up, swirl me around and I would have an overwhelming feeling of relief that it was all over. I honestly thought I would be skipping out of the consultant's office singing happy tunes and feeling like I would live forever. Instead, my reality was a phone call late in the day, where instead of saying "you are cancer free," they explained that from the histology taken from Agnes they could not see any "sign of cancer". They could not see any sign of cancer but they could not guarantee that it was gone and that it would not return. My reality was hardly movie-worthy. On the funny side, can you imagine my oncologist's face if I had been with him in person and I started to run towards him, ready to launch myself into his arms? I am 5ft 10in, two stone overweight and I am sure it's not the done thing to hug anyone in your medical team. Perhaps it was better I got a phone call instead.

As well as the dark shadow behind me, I also have huge guilt that my treatment was a success. I am one of the lucky ones and I worry that I may come across as ungrateful for my outcome when I am not dancing about celebrating. I know others who were going through similar treatment at the same time who never heard any positive news since their diagnosis, and some of those are no longer here. Instead of life being a bed of roses post-treatment I have huge guilt and anxiety. Everyone around me is celebrating and are relieved the problem has passed. I can visibly see friends breathing a sigh of relief that I am no longer sick. I know it was hard to see me fighting my way through treatment and for many it made them feel uncomfortable. I am, however still suffering in the aftermath of such a journey. Everyone else around me has moved on and many expect me to do so too. I can see their discomfort if I mention my struggles and so I try not to say anything. But the scars are deep and I really need to talk about it.

Anxiety

People can say stupid things and I noticed that a lot when I was going through treatment. It seems it doesn't stop when treatment is over, as I had someone tell me to "be grateful and forget cancer ever happened". Simple advice from someone who has not walked in my shoes. Is this what PTSD feels like? I feel in a constant state of shock and worry that the cancer will return. My reality is that medical support continues, with check-ups, blood tests and infusions. My anxiety levels increase every day. I know I am one of the lucky ones, but that does not mean I don't feel the way I am feeling right now. It's hard to forget cancer when right now the chances of it returning are relatively high.

There has been a handful of people who feel they have the right to remind me that I need to be thankful if I mention I am worried that the black shadow of cancer is close. The same people who immediately dismiss my feelings. I am sure it is because it is uncomfortable for them to hear. People tell me "not to worry", but how do you turn off worry and anxiety? You can't. Simple to say, impossible to do. I wrote about hating platitudes in my first book, and being told not to worry as a solution is another useless thing to say, despite me knowing it is always said with kindness.

KINDLY BLUNT MESSAGE

Please don't assume that someone like me is in a daily celebration of survival and that life now feels like one big party. Be kind and know that it will take time to recover from the shock and trauma that cancer and treatment puts people through. Don't try to tell anyone to be happy and move on, as it is far from being as simplistic as that. Instead give them the freedom to talk and, if they want to, time to share how they are feeling.

Over the next five years I will have many check-ups, and so far each one comes with its own buildup of anxiety. I have always thought I was a strong person, but since completing my cancer treatment I think I have PTSD. My type of cancer has a high recurrence rate and that weighs heavily at the back of my mind, a shadow lurking. A dark shadow that is ready to pounce when I least expect it to. I worry every time I have an ache or pain that it might be cancer returning. I am triggered every time I return to the hospital where I had my treatment. It is a place that saved my life and was excellent in everything it did for me, but being back on the ward has me in tears. Seeing sick people still going through treatment hurts deeply, as I know how hard it is and I have huge guilt as a survivor. When I am on the ward I do my best to smile at everyone I see to give them some sort of emotional support. I know I would have appreciated that when I was going through it. Cancer really is shit.

KINDLY BLUNT ADVICE

You can't turn off worry like a light switch, but you can try to distract yourself and live each moment the best you can. When I feel guilty about surviving I think about those that were not as fortunate. I want to live a full life in their honour. They were not given the chance I was given. Cancer feels like a black shadow that is always biting at your ankles. Don't let cancer have the satisfaction of getting the upper hand. You may always have a shadow behind you, but keep the sun in your face as you live life to the full, smile every day and know that it is OK to not feel grateful and happy all of the time. I certainly didn't.

I have no idea if what I am going through is PTSD, and perhaps at this point in my journey I should have sought help from my GP, but I feel like I should be able to bounce back. After being told I was free from cancer, no formal counselling was offered, although I know if I had asked my GP he would have tried to help. But I didn't ask, as I feel I should be grateful the cancer is gone and I don't want to be a bother.

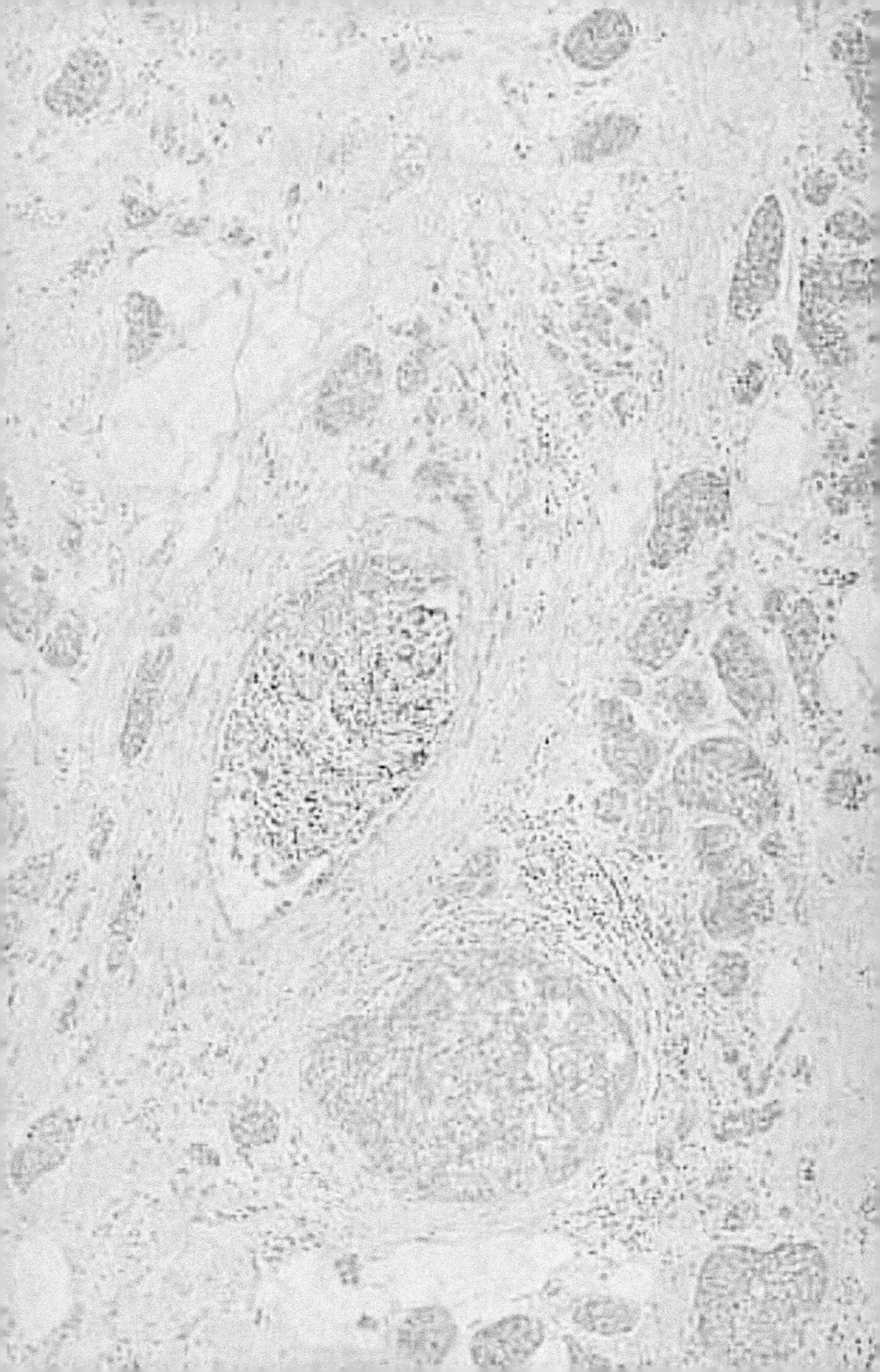

What A Difference A Year Makes

TO CUT A LONG STORY SHORT

"No fear, as I knew there was nothing wrong"

Happy Diagnosis Day

Today is a significant day, it is a year since my diagnosis day. I am not sure I should really call it a "Happy" Diagnosis Day, but I suppose I can call it what I want. Today it is a year since I was told, "I am sorry, you have cancer." Words that have echoed in my head ever since. A year ago today, I jumped in my car and set off for a call back appointment after a routine mammogram. I was carefree, with no worries in the world. The recall letter informed me that four out of 100 people get called back and it was usually not cancer. "Of course it wasn't cancer," I told myself. The idea of me having cancer was ridiculous. So off I went, on my own, for more tests, with the confidence that it would be nothing.

I arrived at my appointment calm and collected, ready to have more tests to show there was nothing seriously wrong. It was lockdown, so it was a short sit in the waiting room with other ladies, all separated by chairs with "Do not sit here" signs. I had no fear at all, as I knew there was nothing wrong. Unfortunately, you will have guessed, that was not the case and after walking into the consultant's room to see my mammogram on the screen, I could see there was a problem. In complete denial I told the consultant it "didn't look good", expecting her to correct me with my amateur scan reading. Unfortunately she agreed with me and that's when it all kicked off, like a nightmare opening up all around me. Soon the team were wheeling in trolleys for biopsies to be taken and an urgent referral to St Lukes Cancer Hospital. To cut a long story short, a story that is in my first book *Agnes, Bea, Cancer and Me*, after more testing over the next few weeks finally I was given the devastating diagnosis of Stage 3 triple negative breast cancer, with spread of that cancer into my axillary lymph nodes. I was in total shock, things like this didn't happen to me. But, in reality, they did.

Last year was the longest year of my life, although today, a year on, it seems like a lifetime away. I had 16 chemotherapy sessions over 21 weeks that saved my life, but literally broke both my body and spirit. Thankfully it also broke cancer and after a unilateral mastectomy and full lymph clearance operation in February 2022, I was given the all-clear. *No sign of cancer in the breast tissue.* The odds of it coming back are in my favour - 60/40, but that still seems high. However, I have decided to live every day to the full. I am going to do my best not to sit around worrying that the cancer will return. Instead I will focus on making great life experiences and to continue running my business that I love.

Today I shall be celebrating as a happy survivor day!

KINDLY BLUNT REMINDER

It can be so easy to get caught up in daily life and let the days pass us by. It can also be really easy to be living a life we don't really like, wishing it was different. Don't be the person that is passing every precious day unhappy and wishing for more. Step up for what you want and go get it. It may not happen overnight, but it can happen if you commit to what you want. Whatever you do, smile every day.

The Guilt Is Strong

It is December 2022 and I am back for my second infusion of zoledronic acid. I had my bloods done a few days ago and got a call to say all is well so I can go ahead with my second infusion. Just like the last infusion, it is hard being back in hospital. I don't think I will ever get used to arriving back on the ward with so many people fighting to stay alive. The guilt is strong today as it is so unfair that many will not get the second chance I am getting to continue living. The smell, the sounds, the familiarity of the cancer unit makes it uncomfortable as emotions around having chemotherapy come flooding back. I have come alone today, as I feel I should be strong enough to do this on my own. It's hard to keep leaning on people and expecting them to support me. I told Eddie I didn't need him to accompany me in a flippant, "this is nothing" type of tone. Now I wish he was here.

KINDLY BLUNT ADVICE

Ask for help when you need it. I made the mistake of putting on the tough exterior that I could do things alone, as after all most people expect me to be fully recovered. On reflection this is not what I should have done. This advice is for anyone that needs some help. Don't be frightened to ask, as most people will be more than happy to step in to support you. If you are supporting someone, don't forget to ask if they still need your support.

Today, I struck up a conversation with a lovely lady in her 70s in the chair next to me who has ovarian cancer. This is the second time she has had to fend off cancer. She had been given the all-clear just a few months ago and was feeling well. She describes how shocked she was to find out it had returned in such a short time. My heart feels heavy listening to her, but I am in awe of how upbeat she is. She wants to reach 80, she tells me. I tell her my next challenge is to get to 60. We chatted about our children and how it was upsetting to worry them with our health battles. My wish is that she gets back to remission. No one should go through chemotherapy, let alone have to do it all again a second time. Cancer, however, does not keep count of how hard it was the first time or care who it lets get through it or not. I hate cancer and the destruction it puts on everyone involved.

In just over an hour I am out of the ward, zoledronic acid circulating in my bloodstream, and walking back to the car. I shed a few tears in relief that it is done and also at the reminder that this is still a big part of my life. Another four infusions to go before I can stop coming here. I am however, truly grateful that for now I appear to be free from any signs of cancer. I intensely know how lucky I am.

It is the day after my infusion and I am boarding a flight to America. I decided that if I had to go into hospital I would do something nice afterwards. I think this may become a thing moving forward. I have my next infusion in June and I think I will be booking another flight after that visit too. I am so grateful I get to do this, a trip away to meet with a business mastermind group I am part of. I am sitting here, in an upgraded seat (who knew economy plus would be so good?), I don't have anyone in the seat next to me and all I can do is smile. There are side effects to the infusion, but no worse than flu-like symptoms for a day or so. The steward comes down the aisle and I order a glass of wine as a way of celebrating and to help me fall asleep. This is me living life.

A YEAR ON

"Hangover football is a moment in time that I will treasure"

I Feel Like No One Cares

No one cares. I am sure they do but I feel alone. Today it is a year since my last chemotherapy session. So many key dates from a year ago. Well, strictly it's not exactly a year, as tomorrow is Christmas Eve but it is Friday 23rd and I used to go on a Friday, so today I am celebrating the end of all that shit. A year ago Percy PICC (the line in my arm to administer chemo and take bloods) was removed and I have a small scar as a reminder of living with it for so long.

I feel like no one cares. Of course, I know Eddie, my children and closest friends care, but it does feel like everyone else has moved on. I suppose until you go through it, you can't understand how terrible that time was and how it has left deep scars both mentally and physically. Last year I was hardly able to walk a few steps and my body was a mess. Today I am off for a walk with friends, something I could only imagine last year. This time last year I could not make the Christmas walk; instead, I struggled to walk 50 yards from the car park to the coffee shop to meet them when they had finished their hike. Today I managed the whole walk, in the pouring rain and it feels fantastic. As I walk, I share with someone that today is a special day for me, but I am quickly dismissed and get told I should forget about it now. This time last year I was near suicidal and my body was broken, and it's impossible to forget. I have spent the past year feeling like I have PTSD, but only sharing those feelings with a few who don't shut me down. Others expect me to be back to normal and never mention the word "cancer" again. If only it was that easy, but it was such a large part of my life and a trauma that still haunts me. People don't expect me still to be in total shock that I had to fight so hard to save my own life. I can't of course, expect people to know how it feels to be a year on, but it would be nice if people let me say openly how I feel, especially when they ask "How are you?"

I know that I am being unreasonably hard on those around me and, really, why should they care. However, cancer is always in my mind, forever in the background, threatening to return. It seems human nature makes people assume it is all over and many are quick to change the subject if I dare to voice my fears.

KINDLY BLUNT ADVICE

In my last book I talked a lot about the importance of listening to help support people going through cancer treatment. I honestly think as humans the biggest gift we can give anyone is giving them a safe place to speak. Be an ear to listen without judgement or advice. I found holding in my worries exhausting and trying to shut up and forget it ever happened was near impossible. I just wanted to be heard rather than shut down. Be the person that listens.

Let Me See Another Christmas

It is Christmas Eve and I am late putting up the tree. I used to love putting the tree up when the children were little and lived at home, but now my nest is empty and without the children the excitement is not quite the same. I find it a chore doing it alone, so it is not unusual that I am doing it at the last minute. I am, however, excited that I have made it to another Christmas, a year ago I was not so sure this would happen. I had hoped that by now I would be back to myself, but it's been a hard year waiting for my body to recover. Wounds have healed well since the mastectomy nine months ago and I have been working hard to rehab the area. I can now do press-ups from my knees, walk five miles at a steady pace and get up off the floor with ease. I am finding losing weight hard despite eating well, it is so slow. I still can't wear many of my clothes and I am getting so fed up wearing a prosthetic boob. Last year at Christmas I had another three months to wait for my mastectomy and for the tissue removed (Agnes and Larry and all the other lymph nodes) to be tested for any sign of cancer. As I get out the decorations to hang on the tree, I vividly remember putting them away last year. I held onto each of my beautiful angel decorations and asked each one to let me see another Christmas. I hoped beyond hope that I would be unwrapping them again to celebrate another Christmas and today that has become a reality. Last year I had no idea if the chemotherapy had worked until I had surgery and the tissue removed tested. Here I am a year later, still alive. As I pull those very same angel decorations out of the box, I thank each and every one of them for letting me live. As I hang them on the tree I feel immense relief and gratitude. One of the angels was given to me by a friend, who after over 10 years was taken by breast cancer. In her honour I hang her angel in the centre of the tree. I realise that I am so fortunate to be one of the lucky ones. I am totally overwhelmed that I have made it and I will never take being alive and well for granted. Each day is a gift and I will live every extra day to the full in honour of those that were not as fortunate as me. Happy Christmas from me and all my angels.

What A Difference A Year Makes

When I couldn't go out during chemo because of the risk of catching Covid, I continually wished I could go out. Now I am well, I find it hard to step confidently out of the door. I look very different, with my wild chemo curls and a body that is too large for my old body shape clothes. But it is New Year's Eve and I am off out. I have lost a bit of weight and tonight I am dressed up in a red and black, floaty, poppy-covered dress with heels and lippy on. I have a new feeling that I have not felt for years. I feel a glimmer of the Helen before all of this. My hair is longer, although it has a lot of growing to do; it has a life of its own and refuses to be tamed. I now sport a full-on cockapoo style. I have done my best to dress up, but there is still an overwhelming sense of being "Helen who had cancer"; Helen who is a survivor but who underneath is shit-scared that her cancer may return. Fortunately, Eddie grabs my hand and we head out the door, despite my best efforts to tell him I would rather be in bed with my head of curls under the duvet.

I realise that a year ago I was still recovering from my last session of chemotherapy and I certainly did not feel pretty. I remember going to a dinner party with friends. I had to buy a large shirt and stretch trousers to fit my larger body. I did throw on a pair of pink stilettos and painted my nails to match, which helped, but I spent the whole evening avoiding being in any of the photos taken. I felt too large, I was bald, at only a week since my last chemo sessions with all that brings, and at that point I had no idea if my cancer was gone. What a difference a year makes. I am a year on after a successful mastectomy operation and a "no sign of cancer" outcome. This time last year I was so frightened about the year ahead. Did I still have cancer? What would the mastectomy be like, would I need radiotherapy, or worse, more chemotherapy? It was hard to look forward to the year ahead. This year is different. I feel hopeful, with a splash of scared in the background with regard to my future. I put on a large smile as we walk into the party.

Alive Happy And Hopeful

It is New Year's Day and Eddie is playing in the annual football match. This should be called hangover football. Eddie has taken the car and I have walked the three miles to find him. I am doing everything to get my fitness back and walking is great exercise. I sit on a bench with my flask of coffee and watch the game. It's great to see a bunch of old friends still playing football. Don't tell them I call them old, but the average age was probably about 65. It was one of the best games of football I have ever watched. The mis-kicks, the long stops when people landed on the floor and the overall fun and camaraderie the men were having. Hangover football is a moment in time that I will treasure. I feel alive, happy and hopeful. It makes me think about life and how I have been guilty of taking for granted the simple but amazing things that happen. I have missed some of the beauty of moments around me. Another prompt from the universe for me to pay attention to life rather than just travel through it. I thought of a new book title today – "Smile Your Way to Success" and I am going to start writing it.

KINDLY BLUNT ADVICE

Make a conscious effort to notice all the positive things you have in your life, not forgetting the small things. It can be easy to overlook everyday things that we all take for granted and miss living the life that is passing us by. None of us know what is around the corner, so make sure you celebrate every minute of your life and enjoy it as you go. Don't forget to smile too.

PLASTIC SURGEON

"I hope Bea is not offended"

99 Percent Sure

When I had my mastectomy and lymph node clearance, I was told I would have the option to have deep inferior epigastric perforator reconstruction surgery at a later date. DIEP, for short, refers to the blood vessels used in the procedure. As they were unsure at that time if the cancer had all gone, they advised against doing the mastectomy and the reconstruction at the same time. As it turned out, when Agnes was removed she had no sign of cancer left and neither did my lymph nodes, but it was a risk none of us were willing to take.

I wasn't sure what reconstruction really meant, because at the time all I focused on was getting rid of Agnes and her cancer cells. My original surgeon had told me I would have to wait a year for more surgery and we agreed I could think more about it then. It is now over a year since my mastectomy to remove Agnes and my referral for further reconstructive surgery has come through. Today, I am in the car with Eddie by my side, driving to a new hospital, a specialist centre for plastic surgery which was set up way back in 1863 as a cottage hospital and, due to its success treating the burns of airmen during World War Two, it became a centre of excellence.

This hospital is recognised as a specialist reconstructive surgery centre for the South East of England. Although this is a specialist centre, and I feel very fortunate to live in a country that has a health system that funds it all, I am not yet convinced I want more surgery. I have been told the recovery from DIEP surgery is at least 12 weeks and right now I am not confident my cancer won't return imminently. I am unsure if I am willing to use up 12 weeks of what could be my shortened life on more hospital visits and the obvious discomfort of recovery. I have no confidence that I will not get sick again and losing 12 precious weeks on recovery is a risk I need to think about carefully.

Eddie and I agree I should at least go and talk to the surgeon. At this point I am adamant that I don't want to go through anymore surgery, but here I am on the way to find out more about it to make an informed decision. I spend the whole journey telling Eddie I am 99 percent sure I won't be having the reconstruction. I don't want to go through major surgery again with drains, stitches and all the anxiety that goes with it. As far as I am concerned, this is a visit that will do no more than confirm I am done with having surgery.

As with every medical appointment, I find myself in a waiting room wishing the minutes would go past faster. Finally it is my turn to see the consultant. We walk into the room to find a lovely lady sitting at her desk, all smiles, and her medical team are the same. Immediately I feel at ease, but as she tells me what it all involves, my mind goes into meltdown. I smile as she talks and, as is my usual default, I make daft comments as she speaks, trying to make light of everything. My internal voice is telling me to shut up, but externally I am babbling away, a protective mechanism when I am nervous. I even use the same joke I used with my previous surgeon about having a needlework sampler on the wall to help me assess her stitching ability. She smiles kindly, but I am sure she was not amused or worse, not sure what the hell I was talking about.

With every medical examination I am asked to strip down and today is no different. Once again I undress for more people to look at Bea, my scar where Agnes once sat and today, my belly too. The consultant plastic surgeon, her assistant and a nurse, as my chaperone, are all gathered around the treatment couch waiting to look at me in detail. At this point, I really don't care who looks at my body, as it has long felt like it belongs to the medical team rather than me. I have lost count of the people who have looked at and photographed me for medical purposes. I am of course very grateful and they are all very kind and follow strict protocol, but even so I feel like a piece of meat lying on the butcher's slab. A tape measure is used as the consultant plastic surgeon measures Bea. She reports to the note taker of the team, "Left side, remaining breast, stage 2 droop." Poor Bea, she didn't get her cell division wrong like Agnes, who had to be removed, yet she now gets an insult about her positioning. I hope Bea is not offended, as she does not deserve this even if she is well into her 50s. I hope she understands at her age it is no surprise. Internally I am a little shocked at the straight-talking medical speak, but I also think it is funny. Little did I know that there were more comical insults to come.

Plenty!

Next it is my stomach's turn to be looked at. The consultant gently takes hold of my belly stretched by my two lovely children and with stretch due to my love of good food. She holds it firmly and gives it a shake. She turns to the team and announces, "There is plenty." This time I can't help but giggle outwardly, as I am well aware I have "plenty" of belly to use to reconstruct a boob. I could supply a few boobs with my belly if they need me to donate. I feel a rush of hilarity, shock and embarrassment all rolled into one. It's amazing how in a medical setting it's normal to say things that if anyone else uttered they would get a stern look. How incredible is science and surgery that they can take my baby belly, which I am now so glad I grew and nurtured, and move that tissue to my chest wall to reconstruct another boob where Agnes once sat. I may have just been insulted but all in good faith and for a valid reason.

Things get interesting as the consultant starts to tell me that, whilst I have the DIEP reconstruction, Bea with her stage 2 droop, can have an uplift to match the new perkier boob they propose to construct. It gets even better when she informs me my belly will also get a full tummy tuck, and while she is in that area she will repair my abdominal muscles which were torn when I was pregnant. In an instant, my thoughts of surgery are changing and now my head is spinning. Oh my goodness, I could have a full make over. I have never wanted any type of plastic surgery and would never have wished to have a nip and tuck to change the way I looked. I just wanted to grow older and look the best I could for my age as I went. However, right now it feels like there are some benefits of surgery: a new boob, a hitched-up, perky Bea, a tummy tuck and abdominal muscle repair. Perhaps I could have a new career in granny modelling after this? After all, I am good at being photographed for hospital records.

The consultant is kind and listens carefully as I explain my fear of spending 12 weeks in recovery. She reassures me that the recovery time, although 12 weeks, is mostly advice not to lift heavy things during that period. No hoovering, using the washing machine, lifting shopping bags. This is getting better and better. I will be able to walk straight away and that gives me a lot of comfort. My mind is spinning. I thought I would go into this meeting, listen and then say, "No thank you," but now there are options that I do need to consider.

We get back in the car and I feel sad as the tears flow. I could fill a reservoir with all the crying I do lately. I should feel elated that I can have reconstruction or relieved that I won't be going through it, but my head is a mush, I am so confused. What do I do? Eddie patiently listens as he drives me home. I am going back and forth as I try to work out what to do. Finally, as is his way, he tells me I don't have to decide yet. I can stay on the surgery list and I can pull out anytime I wish. Poor Eddie, he has been through so much being my support. I do think his ears must feel like they are bleeding at times with the amount of moaning I do. Today he is due to be on a pub crawl with his mates and he declined the boys' outing to accompany me. We have finished the appointment earlier than we anticipated, so I tell him I will drop him off at the brewery his mates have stopped at. At least he can have some fun and smiles today after being with me.

Unusually, I decide I don't want to go straight home so I stop at a local pub for lunch. I would really like to talk to a friend about this, but asking for support is so hard. I should call someone but it feels impossible. It is not in my DNA to ask for help and I have worried people enough since my diagnosis. Instead, I sit alone trying to make sense of my change of mindset and try desperately to work out what is best for me. Luckily I am sitting in a booth so I can hide the tears that are flowing yet again. I thought things were supposed to get easier, but I still feel I am in whirlwind of decisions with regard to my health. A roller coaster that keeps throwing up new twists and turns.

Poor Bea

It's a week since I went to the specialist hospital and I have just received a letter from my plastic surgeon, which is an overview about where I am in my treatment. How odd that I now talk about "my plastic surgeon". I feel like a celebrity who is having a nip and tuck to keep their looks. I never imagined I would have plastic surgery. The letter has the usual "nice-to-meet-you" type of introduction, but my eyes are quickly drawn to the next paragraph. The words jump out of the page at me. "You have a grade 2 ptosis (sagging) of your left breast." I nearly spat out my coffee at the word "sagging" written in brackets. As a retired osteopath, I understand what ptosis means, but I understand many patients may not. It is official, Bea is "sagging". No surprise, but still strange to see it in writing. Who knew boobs were graded according to how much they sag? Poor Bea, I hope she didn't realise I was laughing at her predicament. The good news is she will get a surgical lift if I go through with the DIEP reconstruction. A Bea facelift, I wonder if she will appreciate it or if she is happy with her current sag? If you have boobs or one boob like me, did you just look down and try to work out what grade you would be after reading this?

The letter continues to inform me that I need to have a CT angiogram. A DIEP reconstruction uses the fat from the stomach area to create a new boob shape and for that tissue to survive they need to do microsurgery to connect it to blood vessels in the reconstruction area. If I am to have surgery they need to check the blood vessels in my abdomen are good enough to have a chance of the surgery being successful. I need to wait until I get sent that appointment before we can go any further. More testing, but it is what I need to do if I do decide to go back under the surgeon's knife. I wish I knew with some certainty what I was going to do, but right now I am just focusing on getting the tests done before I make an informed decision.

KINDLY BLUNT ADVICE

Embrace your body as it is right now. How often do you berate yourself for the odd bulge? If you are striving for that perfect body whilst missing the point that you have an amazing body that supports you quite literally in everything you do, then please stop. Instead of judging your body against your idea of perceived perfection, why not treat your body well instead? Feed it well, hydrate it and move it as much as you can. Your body deserves more than you looking in a mirror daily and criticising it. Instead, look after it. Your body deserves you to treat it well. Your body is bloody amazing and so are you.

Thank You For Being My Therapist

I like to journal daily and it gives me comfort to note how I feel. Journaling has become my own form of therapy and as I find it impossible to ask for support it has been an important part of my recovery. Everyday I write "every cell in my body is healthy and cancer free". In reality this is unlikely to reduce the chances of the cancer returning, but I have nothing to lose by doing it. More importantly, it makes me feel good even if it is done with a touch of desperation.

Today I have decided to ring the support centre at the cancer unit as I really feel I need to talk things through with a mental health expert. My anxiety levels are off the scale and I want help to put the dark thoughts behind me. The centre offers free support for people going through cancer. However, when I was in the process of going through treatment the last thing I wanted to do was go back to the hospital on yet another day. I was already there at least twice a week. During it all I wanted to push through the treatments and my focus was solely on that. I didn't go for the NHS makeup sessions, relaxing treatments or the counselling as I just did not have the capacity for that as well as receiving treatment. I understand that many people need support during the treatment time, but I was not ready for it at that time. Post-cancer diagnosis and treatment, the shock of it all came out and for me it was many months after I had finished treatment. I had extreme anxiety about the cancer returning, I had lost my self worth, my business had suffered, my body image was on the floor, I had severe menopause symptoms and the huge guilt of being a survivor. It has taken a lot of courage for me to phone the centre, but when I speak to the receptionist she tells me I am too late to use any of their services. It is over a year from my last chemo treatment, so that means I am no longer eligible to receive any support despite never using their services previously. She suggests I call my GP and ask for help but after receiving a straight "no" from the support centre I have shut down and I will not be asking anyone for help again. This may not be the most sensible option, but I am a proud person and this is the option I choose.

I wrote my book *Agnes, Bea, Cancer and Me* as a form of therapy and now this book is going to help me too. I want to thank you for listening and being my therapist as I work my way through the unknown.

Let Loose To Sail Alone

A few days after the New Year celebrations I am due a routine call from the oncologist. I don't wait around for medical phone calls anymore as they are often not on time. I am too busy living life to waste time waiting, so when my phone rings I am out on a walk with my good friend Jackie. I recognise the hospital number easily as it is the telephone number that calls me the most these days. Instead of hearing the voice of my oncologist it is his secretary and she explains she has good news. Moving forward, I no longer need to speak to my oncologist consultant (Mr K). Instead the oncology team will be in charge of my care. I am being signed off from my oncologist's main list.

I finish the call and relay the good news to Jackie, but deep inside me it strangely doesn't seem like good news. This man saved my life, I trusted my life with him and he came good on his pledge to rid me of the cancer. But it feels like my lifeline has been cut and I feel intense concern that I am no longer under Mr K's care. I have hung my hopes off his every word and trusted him to lead me through the worst of times. He truly is a superhero in my eyes and I feel scared that he is no longer overseeing everything. I keep telling myself it is a good thing, as he only hangs around if there is cancer about and he has signed me off from his personal care. I should be happy, but I have feelings of being let loose to sail alone and I have no idea if I am safe. The ties have been cut, the regular visits and reassuring chats have stopped. The man that sent me for so much chemotherapy should be someone I am glad to see the back of, but he was my safety net. I felt safe with him being in control of my care; he also was one of the only people on the medical team that made me belly-laugh at the worst of times. It's an odd feeling, as this man saved my life and yet I should be celebrating never seeing him again. I have mixed emotions, but I remind myself that although it is scary, it is very good news. I imagine he could be dancing around his office, dressed in his superhero cape, celebrating not having to put up with my weird sense of humour and constant moaning at every visit moving forward. Secretly I hope he is happy and does slightly miss me.

Mr K, if you read this, I want to publicly thank you for saving my life. For helping me live longer, giving my husband his wife back, allowing my kids to have their mum present at their weddings and for being the most incredible human being. You made me laugh when times were hard and you were empathetic to the tough journey I was on when it mattered. You are and always will be my superhero. THE BIGGEST THANK YOU from me and all the other people you continue to help every day.

SHOW AND TELL

"Why do I I have so many worries when I am cancer free?"

Brave Women

I still recoil when I see a medical letter arrive on my door mat. My mind automatically assumes it will be bad news. I was going to say it's a totally irrational feeling, but I have had so many letters ranging from devastating news to celebratory news that it's understandable I dislike the regularity that medical letters still get posted through my letterbox.

It's a day for medical appointments today. I have got a second letter inviting me to an event at the plastic surgery hospital. I shall describe it as "show and tell". I have been invited to meet other women who have had the DIEP operation. Of course, this is not going to be a "show and tell" like in school where you took your favourite toy to show the class. Instead, I will be seeing brave women showing the results of their surgery. I want to go to this event so I can listen and talk to women who have real experience of the operation. It sounds like I am going to meet some amazing women. I hope this event will help me make up my mind as to whether I should go ahead with reconstruction. I am intrigued to see and hear about other people's experiences.

Today we are back at the specialist hospital for the show and tell plus Q&A session. Partners are allowed in for the first part, where a nurse is telling us all about it. As I look around, I notice that there are a lot of women that look like me. Short and very curly hair is the general look for at least half of the women in this room. I realise they are post-treatment and their similar hair regrowth and curls mean we all had treatment around the same time. Not everyone has had cancer in the room, however, some people have the BRCA gene mutation and I realise they are here for preventative breast surgery and reconstruction.

For modesty, the men in the room are asked to leave after the talk from the nurse. I laugh internally as I imagine Eddie inside the hospital's men creche. I call out after him as he is led out of the room, "Don't worry, I will come and collect you at home time." At the front of the room are eight women of varying ages, who bravely share their stories and their scars. I am so inspired by each and every one of the women and it makes me consider the reconstruction surgery more seriously. Of course, I am only hearing from those who had positive outcomes, but their stories are compelling and they all look fabulous. One lady shares that she is glad she had it done because she no longer looks in the mirror and thinks about cancer. Her comment triggers something in me. I want that feeling. I want to get up, get dressed without a thought for cancer. Will that ever be possible?

Thirty minutes later I set off to collect Eddie from the man creche. He has had a fabulous time with the other men at the event and a lady volunteer who has been through the DIEP procedure. They have been discussing the details of the operation and the expected recovery. They had also been discussing, much to my surprise, my book *Agnes, Bea, Cancer and Me*. Eddie had told them all about it and as the men filtered out the room past me, I had comments of "Well done" and "Amazing". The lady volunteer wanted to know where she could get the book. I have decided that Eddie is now head of my book marketing team, just don't tell him as it is an unpaid role.

Engaged

Good things do still happen and today I have extra to celebrate. I have just heard from my daughter that she has got engaged. We had a heads-up from her now fiance but it was lovely to hear the proposal was a success. I am so happy for her and her future husband, a great guy who we love and who loves her lots. What a great start to my day hearing the news. The news, however, makes me reflect on my health. Good news, but I am worrying again about cancer returning. My son is getting married in October this year and my daughter gets married next year. I have to stay well. I don't want to spoil their day with any worry or drama that I would cause if I got ill again. Why do I have so many worries when I am cancer free? This is not how I imagined life after the dreaded C. When you see it on the TV those that get the "all-clear" skip off into the sunset with their life returning to normal in an instant. Unfortunately this is not reality and it is going to take a bit longer, but today I have fabulous news and I am going to smile all day.

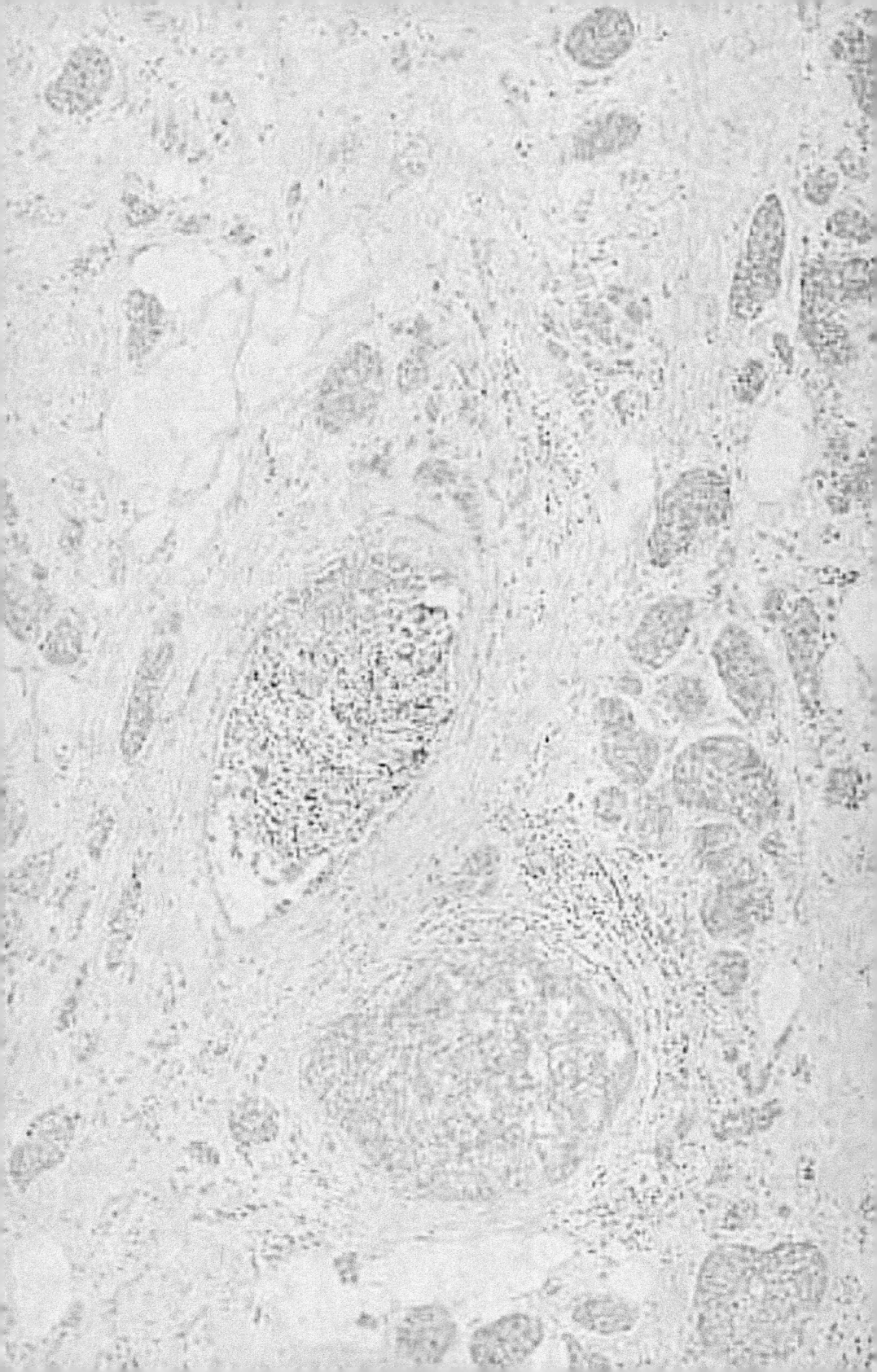

Fuss Over Nothing

LOSING MY SENSE OF REALITY

"Every cell in my body is healthy and cancer free"

I Am Not Frightened Of Death

Panic is a regular emotion post-cancer. Every little ache or pain I immediately think is cancer that has come back. The hospital team have told me to be vigilant, as triple negative breast cancer commonly reoccurs in the first few years after treatment. The word vigilant makes me feel the seriousness of my situation.

I started a cold a few weeks ago and it has not subsided. Even Eddie starts to ask if I should go back to see the GP. Of course, I should be rushing back to the medics to get checked, but I worry that they will think I am making a fuss. A fuss about nothing, but what if it is not? My cough won't ease and I am having trouble swallowing. Not being able to swallow prior to cancer would make me think I have a simple throat infection, but today my mind goes straight to throat cancer. I jump to worst-case scenario without any evidence. I call the GP surgery and immediately they are very keen to see me, which is good but somewhat disconcerting. My worry is now off the scale but I am reluctant to go as they may confirm my worst fears and tell me I have cancer again. How will I cope a second time?

I am called in to see a GP I have not seen before. I am a keen supporter of the medical profession and perhaps it is because I am anxious, but this GP almost instantly makes me mad. She is disorganised and doesn't seem to have a handle on who I am or my medical background. It is obvious she has not looked at my notes prior to me walking in the door. I was an osteopath for many years and I always checked patients' notes before seeing them, and I expect the same when I am seen. I fully understand that I used to have more time than a GP, but I should not have to update her on my cancer background. In my head I am screaming, "Look at your notes, I am at risk of cancer returning and I want you to acknowledge my worry." Of course I don't scream at her and, despite being mad at her, she finally does seem to pull it together to do some examinations of my mouth and lungs. I am soon leaving with a prescription for oral thrush and a new steroid inhaler, as she thinks my asthma has flared up. I agree with her about the asthma but not thrush. I had oral thrush during my chemotherapy and this does not feel the same. I should have questioned her on this, instead, I am just glad to get out of her disorganised office. Perhaps I should have stayed and offered to tidy up for her, or even better, realise that everyone can have a bad day and perhaps this was hers.

The day after the GP, despite feeling under the weather, I head out to do battle ropes and two short runs. I am on a fitness challenge and I don't want to miss today's session. It is freezing outside and it's hard to take a breath. I do, however, manage to plod along at a slow pace but, I know my chest is limiting me and that I shouldn't even be exercising today. I am finding it difficult to breathe and, to my horror, it's pronounced on my right side. Now my head goes into overdrive. I already think the discomfort swallowing is more on the right side and now it feels like the top of my right lung is restricted. The right side is where Agnes and her cancer used to sit. I have pathological knowledge as a retired osteopath, so you can imagine my brain going over all the worst possibilities, which is as bad as googling health symptoms. My brain loses all sense of reality and jumps again to the worst-case scenario. I now think I have an apical tumour of the lung. Did rogue cancer cells migrate there? Is that why I can't shift this cough? Right now I have no idea what is going on, but I do know that I am worried enough to make contact with my breast cancer nurse. Time to get the big guns involved. The disorganised GP did not fill me with confidence, so I am going to the specialist team for their opinion.

What strikes me as interesting during this period of anxiety about my health is that I realise that I am not frightened of death. I am, however, scared of having more treatment. I would not wish chemotherapy on my worst enemy and it's unthinkable right now to imagine how I would get through it again. My mind cascades into thoughts of never seeing any future grandchildren and, more pressing, that I could be sick for my son's upcoming wedding or worse, not make it at all. Irrational thinking that means I am now in tears typing an email to my oncology nurse. I don't want to make a fuss, but I also know I have to. The cancer shadow starts to envelop me, threatening to take me to a dark place.

Within a couple of hours, I get a reply from the nurse and I am asked to speak to my GP surgery immediately to get a chest x-ray and a blood screen. The email has a sense of urgency, which does not help my anxiety. A different GP is quick to refer me for the necessary tests and off I go once again to the local hospital. I am thinking I could perhaps do group tours of local hospitals, I have been to so many. Helen's Hospital Tours has a certain ring to it. As always the NHS is brilliant. I am seen quickly and, although the wait seemed like a lifetime, in which I have planned my own funeral and who would have my jewellery when I am gone, they get the results back to me in just a few days. The results show I have a chest infection, missed by the previous GP, that needs antibiotics, but there is no sign of any mass in my lungs or markers raised in my blood screen. Funnily enough, I don't have oral thrush. I make a mental note to never see that GP again.

This is my new mantra: "Every cell in my body is healthy and cancer free." I am keeping focused on that the best I can. Now to get to breathing easily and get on with living my life away from the cancer shadow.

KINDLY BLUNT REMINDER

If you or your loved ones think something is "not quite right", get seen by an expert. You are not wasting their time or making a fuss. They are happy to see you and give you their expert advice.

A Bubbles Sort Of Day

It's March 2023 and I have received a letter calling me in for my first annual check-up. My cancer journey is far from over, as I have to be monitored regularly by the oncology team for at least the next five years. I am thankful, but also hate the reminder that the chance of it returning is real, hence the need for regular check-ups.

Today is my appointment day, and I have arrived in plenty of time, but the consultant is running late. There is a note on the screen that her clinic is running late and as so much time passes Eddie has to go and move the car to avoid a parking ticket. By the time I go in she is an hour late. I can't help but get grumpy when I have to wait. I am trying to live my life and yet to save my life I have to sit wasting precious minutes in a waiting room. Of course, some of the bad mood is brought on by worry that something may be found and today I don't have Eddie to join me in the meeting as she is so late. I walk into the room and I am not being seen by the previous consultant or my oncologist. Instead another lady consultant is sitting at the desk. I am already grumpy that I have had to wait so long, but that mood gets worse as it is apparent she has not even glanced at my notes before I walk in. She comes across as being very disorganised and seems almost as grumpy as me. Call me demanding, but it is important to me that she knows who I am and what I am here for. I also want to feel that she cares in some small way. First impressions are not good, as I feel like an inconvenience to her busy day. Finally, once I update her about my type of cancer etc she is ready to examine me. Unusually, I am not wanting to talk or make the usual witty comments my mind usually conjures up. Instead, I wish I was somewhere else as she carries out a manual examination of Bea and where Agnes used to sit. Aside from my judgement that she has poor bedside manner skills, her examination seems thorough and I soften a little as she tells me everything is as it should be. A wave of relief washes over me and memories of waiting for over an hour disappear in an instant.

I get home and celebrate with a huge glass of champagne. It's become a bubbles sort of day and the relief is immense. Time to keep living life. Woo hoo!

TRIGGERS

"I smile through gritted teeth"

Think Before You Speak

Words are strange things. They can make you laugh, they can make you cry, they can make you sad or even bore you. I was sensitive to other people's words when I went through my chemo and it seems I am still sensitive to words people throw at me now I am on the other side.

I have told a few people that I am thinking about having reconstructive surgery. Agnes has gone and perhaps it is time to replace her? I have not yet made my final decision, but I am busy weighing up the pros and cons. The plan, if I go ahead with it, is to use my tummy fat. Seems a waste not to, as I seem to have perfected the perfect boob on my tummy area over the last 20 plus years. It's almost like I knew to eat more so I had my own ready-made spare body part. Most people I tell are intrigued to learn what the medics can do and how clever the reconstruction process is. The surgeon wants to make sure I have the best results possible. Of course that is obvious, but I am happy the plan is not just going to take a slice off my belly and make an Agnes replacement. She will make sure my abdomen looks the best it can, she spoke of giving Bea a lift (Bea has a stage 2 droop, remember) and, if time permits, repair the split I never knew I had in my abdominal muscles. All this is fascinating to both me and those I tell, but there is a phrase that has been used twice by people when I explain the operation. The words they used were "Mummy Makeover". The first time someone used it I had to look up the meaning. Apparently a "Mummy Makeover" includes breast surgery and a tummy tuck to neaten up a woman's body after having children. Yes, it is a real thing. I have never wanted to cover my stretch marks or get rid of my "Mum Tum". I object strongly to being compared to someone who has surgery to rejuvenate their body after childbirth. Of course, it's subjective and if you want a "Mummy Makeover", go for it, but it was never on my want list. Instead, I am considering reconstructive surgery to repair what cancer treatment has done to my body. With just one boob it's hard to have symmetry unless I wear a prosthetic and the more I live with my current body shape the more I realise I am too lazy to keep wearing a false boob.

People also feel they can give me their advice about my surgery. I often wonder if people actually hear themselves when they say certain things, usually with a smile. One memorable comment, flippantly thrown my way, was, "A tummy tuck is the most painful surgery to have done and it commonly doesn't go to plan." Why would you say that to anyone? Talk about hitting a girl when she is down. I feel my blood rising and steam would be coming out of my ears if I knew how to release the pressure. I smile through gritted teeth and reply, "I am sure if I have got through 16 rounds of chemotherapy and a mastectomy then I can cope with reconstruction surgery." Of course I have no idea if I can get through it, but going on previous performance with this shit journey the odds are looking good in this tough old bird's favour. I don't believe anyone says anything with malice, I just wish they would think just a little before they comment or pass judgement. I am struggling to work out if reconstruction is for me and comments like this are not helpful.

> **KINDLY BLUNT TIP**
>
> I don't want to frighten anyone from speaking to someone who has cancer or is post-cancer. I just want you to think before you speak as being flippant is not going to help them. Instead, listen to their story if they want to talk or respect their wishes if they don't want it mentioned. Rather than comment on something you don't understand listen and learn instead. Certainly never tell anyone the operation they may have is going to be extremely painful.

Right now it's not just words that I am triggered by. Seeing people smoke, drink to excess, eat highly processed food and neglect exercising is a huge trigger for me. I get unreasonably annoyed by people that are taking their health for granted. It seems that many people are prepared to play Russian roulette with their lives. I don't expect people to never have a drink, eat takeaways or have a day on the sofa in their PJ's but I don't understand, since having cancer, why anyone would take a chance with their health. Of course, it is none of my business what others do, but that does not stop me feeling sad when I see someone increasing their chances of getting a major illness by the way they live.

In my reading since having cancer I have learnt that current research suggests, post breast cancer, to drink less than four units of alcohol a week, to do 20 mins of exercise at least three times a week, weight train and to keep weight to normal levels. I believe you should move every day rather than just three times a week. That comes from my experience as a retired osteopath and that is what I aim for. I know that research is only as good as the researcher and methodology used, but I have nothing to lose by following these recommendations. It certainly won't do me any harm.

> **KINDLY BLUNT REMINDER**
>
> Increase your chances of staying healthy. It is good to follow the 80/20 rule. 80 percent of the time you live well and 20 percent you treat yourself. We all have to live and I am never going to give up having the occasional piece of chocolate fudge cake. It's not always possible to give up things you know are detrimental to your health, but there are people out there that can help. See your GP, join a support group and, please, move your body every day.

My Words Were Triggering Too

During feedback on my book *Agnes, Bea, Cancer and Me* I had someone feedback that I should not use the words "fight" or "battle" to describe how I dealt with my cancer journey. They felt this was triggering and disrespectful to those that did not survive cancer. However, in my own defence, I did not use the words "fight" and "battle" to do any more than describe how I felt I get through things. I have always felt I am a fighter, so much so that I used to love Fight Club classes where I actually did punch a bag with my pink boxing gloves. If I was younger I would have loved to have fought in a ring. Virtually fighting is my way of dealing with anything. I understand that words like battle and fight should not be used to describe another person's cancer journey, as not everyone will feel they want to tackle it that way and it can also imply someone wins or loses the battle. I was fighting to get through things on a daily basis. Feeling like a fighter inspired me.

I thought long and hard about whether I should have used the "fight" type words. I concluded that my book was about my personal cancer journey and for that reason I will use whatever words I want. The story in Agnes, Bea, Cancer and Me was my story. I will never suggest that anyone else should use the term "fight", but I needed to approach it in this way. It helped me feel powerful against the unknown. I looked up suggested alternatives, but when I googled it came up with "praying to get through this" which is a problem for me as I am not religious and it is in no way inspiring to me. There was advice that said I should say, "I am thankful I am here," but I didn't feel that would help me get through things. I guess that suggestion was from someone who has never been through it. Of course I was thankful, but I needed more to get through every day. Nothing I found online described how I felt I wanted to deal with cancer. I like to win… is that wrong too? My book never said anyone else had to take on the same mindset as me, in fact, it states it is subjective to my journey and how I wanted to deal with it. I focused on winning and, just like the odds on a lottery, I was just lucky that my outcome was positive. I know it could have been very different and, let's face it, my fight is not over yet. The important thing is that everyone going through a cancer journey should be able to describe it any way they wish. Fight, pray, ignore, scream or any other chosen word can be used if it helps you.

I thought long and hard about taking the apparent triggering words out of my book but they were my words, to help me on my journey and that is why I am proud they stayed in the book.

LIFE-SAVING BINGO

"I think I may have wet myself"

Two Stars

Off to the specialist plastic surgery hospital today. I am having yet another scan. Today it is a computed tomography angiogram, where they are going to scan my abdomen to check whether I've got good enough blood vessels in my stomach to link up with the vessels where Agnes used to sit. Think of it as checking out the pipes before they go ahead with the big plumbing job. I hope I have good plumbing and the pipes are not too rusty.

I arrive in a part of the hospital I have not been to before and I find my way to a waiting room that I can only describe as tatty. Perhaps I am being a little harsh as it is a functional waiting room, but it's very tired. I am seriously thinking of doing a "Patients' Guide to Waiting Rooms" moving forward. I could give them stars and ratings just like hotel accommodation. I'm sure it would catch on. This waiting room would get a two star rating, and that's me being generous. I am in this room on my own with an information board on the wall that is showing there is a 40-minute waiting time. There is no one else around so I wonder how there can be a 40-minute delay. Perhaps I am in the wrong place? So many waiting rooms I could have chosen the wrong one, but there is no one to ask so I stay seated and keep my fingers crossed. Just as I start to panic about where everyone is, another patient walks through the door and sits down. As is done in these places, we both smile sympathetically, I then look down at the floor and she looks down at her phone.

Then I hear the tapping. That irritating noise a phone makes when you have the button sound on. The noise that every normal person turns off or at least I feel they should. She continues tapping and it's like a dripping tap to my brain. Inwardly I roll my eyes, or perhaps I do it outwardly, I am not sure. I hate hospitals, I hate waiting in waiting rooms and I now hate tapping. Seems I am not in a good mental headspace today. After what seems a lifetime of tapping, she gets called through. I love the silence until the realisation that I was here first and I am still waiting. This waiting room and the tapping has turned me into a grump. Actually, cancer has changed me and I don't like being this way.

House

Finally, a friendly nurse appears and I am called through to the CT angiogram machine. I think as a patient you should be given an examination bingo card that a nurse can verify every time you experience yet another type of investigation. I could have shouted "house" by now for completing more than one line, perhaps even the whole card. I am of course thankful that the NHS has been brilliant in my cancer diagnosis and treatment and that the tests I have already had done were beneficial to me. I have had PET scans, MRI scans, nuclear medicine, x-rays, blood tests and I am sure some I have forgotten. No one wants to call "bingo" when it's for having so many tests done, but I am sure I am getting pretty close to shouting "bingo" loudly soon. I have a little word with myself as I lie on the machine bed that I am grateful for all the care and attention I have had. Life-saving bingo is how I shall refer to it in the future. The nurses laugh as I relay my idea to them. I am glad I have found something to amuse me and the team too.

The CT machine is interesting. I am lying with both arms over my head, a cannula has been inserted into my left arm. I am about to have a contrast dye put into my body. This dye helps to show up the blood vessels in my abdomen. The nurses are kind and set me up before leaving the room to start the machine and administer the contrast dye into my body, remotely. It is amazing the technology that humans have invented. The staff are all outside the room and although I can hear them talking to me, I feel incredibly alone. The machine moves me back and forth, in and out of the halo gantry of the scanner. I am thankful this machine does not fully enclose me in. On my bingo card I have had that sort of scan and I don't want to do it again. I get instructions from the machine and then the nurses speak to me and tell me the contrast is going to be given. I have been warned about how the contrast would feel, but when they said it may feel like I am wetting myself, I decided it was unlikely to really feel like that. Silly nurses- surely it would not be like that? How wrong was I. I get a tingling first at the back of my throat, then down my arms and then the warm sensation in my nether regions that really does feel like I have wet myself. After a short while I can hear muffled voices and then the door to the enclosed room I am in is opened. A nurse comes to tell me the machine is not working properly. I still have my arms over my head so I ask if I can move them. I don't quite have full range of movement in my mastectomy side so it has been a struggle keeping my arm in that position. They allow me to rest a while and then they tell me they will start again. I have not had any radiation yet, but I will have to have the contrast given to me again. This time I know it will feel like I have wet myself so I get ready for this very odd experience. We go again and I experience the weird feeling "down there". "Goodness," I think maybe I have wet myself?" I have no idea at this point. It is not long before the CT scan is done and

I am getting myself off the bed. I chat to the nurses and before I know it I have mentioned my book about *Agnes and Bea Cancer and Me*. I also tell them there is a second book and that this story will be in it. I am nothing but true to my word. If you are those nurses and you are reading this - thank you for looking after me so well despite the tech failing for a while. You handled it well, I am also glad I did not wet myself on the second attempt despite thinking I had.

JUST CHECKING

"My brain is doing somersaults as I automatically think the cancer has returned"

Obsessed

I have become obsessed with checking my chest area. This may seem like a good thing considering I am at an increased chance of cancer returning, but checking myself daily, sometimes twice a day, is a constant cancer reminder. I have decided to stop checking myself daily. It has become a negative rather than a positive action, as thoughts of cancer returning increase every time I do it. Instead, I will check myself once a week. A full breast examination including my armpit, chest and neck area. I decide that I won't check on a Friday, as if I did find something I would have to wait all weekend before I could see a specialist. I don't think I could bear the anxiety. I am going to find it hard to leave it to just once a week, but I know that doing it daily is not good for my mental health. It makes me worry, but I like the idea that I am doing it regularly but not daily. I am determined that if this comes back I will be vigilant and catch it as early as possible. I thought being cancer free would make me feel calmer, but in truth I am more worried now than I was before. It feels like I am in the danger zone. The more time passes from that initial all-clear, the more I wonder if my body is recruiting rogue cancer cells that are just waiting to resurface.

KINDLY BLUNT REMINDER

This is a message that I wish I could put on every page of this book. Make sure you check yourself regularly. For a breast examination it is important to also check the armpit and around the neck and collarbone area. Check out this link for full details https://www.cancerresearchuk.org/about-cancer/breast-cancer/symptoms

Concern And Black Shadows

Today my mastectomy scar is uncomfortable. It feels swollen, tight and itchy. Oh god, it doesn't feel right. The scar is where they removed Agnes and all my axillary lymph nodes. It runs across the right side of my chest and curves up into my armpit. On my last hospital visit I was told to be vigilant around the scar, as although the mastectomy took away the breast tissue (aka Agnes) there is no guarantee a few rogue cells were not left. Reading up on the statistics of recurrence in a scar following a mastectomy, with lymph nodes affected, I find one article states it could be as high as 25 percent. I contact my breast cancer team, who immediately make me an appointment with one of the oncology consultants. I am booked in for the next day. I can't fully express how brilliant the NHS has been to me throughout this horrible journey.

My brain is doing somersaults, as I automatically think the cancer has returned. The worry comes and goes over the next 24 hours. I try so hard not to let my mind get too distracted with the what-ifs. My main worry is that my son Joe has his wedding in six months and my daughter Louise has hers next year. I don't want to spoil their special days by being sick again. Worse, my mind wanders to the reality that if cancer has come back then will I see either of their weddings? I know it may seem like I am jumping the gun as I have not had the check-up yet, let alone results, but I defy anyone not to see their life closing in before them when the black shadow of cancer starts closing in. I don't want to spoil my kids' weddings, and I don't want to be a burden and a worry to them. I put them through enough when I went through it the first time. Every parent's nightmare is to impact their children in a negative way.

The next day I sit, with Eddie, in the waiting room waiting to be called in to see the consultant. I am feeling calmer and I have convinced myself that I am making a fuss and that there is nothing wrong. I even start to think I am wasting the medical team's time. It's strange how many of us have these sort of thoughts when we visit the GP or other medical appointments. Thoughts of making a fuss and even regret at asking a medic to check us out. But, as I used to tell my patients when I was a working osteopath, if you are in any doubt, go and see the medics. You are not wasting anyone's time, and getting checked early will, for most conditions, increase your chances of recovery. The best thing that can happen is you have nothing to worry about after being seen and you can relax and feel glad you got things checked out. The medical team you are seeing are being paid to be experts and their job is to check patients every day.

Finally, after a wait, I get called into the consultation room and I explain my symptoms. Instantly I see the concern across the face of the consultant. I was hoping she would dismiss my worries as nothing and I would be on my way. Crap, this feels like the day I got called back after my life-saving mammogram. Instead, she is asking me to undress and she does a full examination of the scar, my armpit and around my clavicle. I expect her to say there is nothing to worry about then but instead she calls the ultrasound clinic and I am sent direct to their waiting room for immediate assessment.

Now I am really worried. I am remembering the recall day way back in 2021 when I had a mammogram that was referred. The memory of arriving clutching a letter that said it would probably be nothing, then being told it was cancer resurfaces to haunt me now. The black shadow is enveloping me and I can feel absolute panic overtaking every part of my body. I feel a tightness in my chest and tears are brewing.

I am now sitting in yet another area of the hospital waiting for an ultrasound. They explain it could be fat necrosis or a return of my cancer. I have never wished for "fat" before, but right now I want it to be anything but cancer. Fat necrosis means death of tissue due to loss of blood supply. The consultant has also felt a lump in the tissue and now my mind is out of control. I am certain it is going to be bad news and I start to work out how I am going to cope with more chemotherapy. My anxiety is heightened as a lady comes out of the scan room and instantly bursts into tears as she tells her husband, "My cancer is back." My heart breaks as she falls into his embrace, sobbing. All of this is far too real. How did I get to be so involved in this cruel world of cancer? I am surrounded by people on the same journey, some with positive outcomes and others who are not so fortunate. It all seems so unfair. Cancer is unfair.

Although it seems like an age I am soon lying on the examination couch with the ultrasound handpiece being run over the area of concern. There is little chit-chat, as for once I don't rattle on about everything and nothing. I physically can't talk right now. I want the sonographer to tell me quickly what I have to deal with. I am convinced it is bad, as there has been very little good news on this journey. However, she won't tell me anything, instead she lets me get dressed and I am sent back to the oncology consultant's waiting area to hear the results. I have another excruciating wait in a packed waiting room until I am taken through to the oncologist. To my relief, she is quick to get to the point and reports I have scar tissue in the area and there is no need for concern. She shares her surprise as she tells me she too thought it was cancer returning. I feel her relief as well as my own.

I think I could have filled multiple swimming pools with the amount of tears I have cried since this all started and today is no different. We get back to the car and the tears flow. Tears of relief, guilt and sorrow for those that are not as fortunate as me. My mind can't get over the lady before me that had a negative outcome and how sad I feel for her and what she will have to face. Guilt is huge when you are as lucky as me. The dark shadow lifts, but it is still right behind me, waiting, and I know I have to be vigilant.

My Story

BOOK LAUNCH

"The reality that I could have died weighs heavy"

Agnes, Bea, Cancer And Me Is Live

Today is book launch day. My first book *Agnes, Bea, Cancer and Me* is live on Amazon and bookshop platforms, and ready to be sent out into the world. It's a big day, and as soon as I share that the book is available to purchase, the sales flood in.

My hope is this book will help others going through the journey of a cancer diagnosis and chemotherapy treatment. I want the book to also support those caring for them and to help anyone who needs help knowing what to say to someone with cancer. I am proud of myself. It's not often I feel that way but today I do. I have made something positive out of my worst nightmare and if it helps others then it is all worth it. My social media has exploded with hundreds of comments from people congratulating me on the book. It is a highly emotional day and one I will never forget. By the end of the day the reality that I could have died weighs heavy. A feeling that I had pushed to the back of my mind, but today it is front and centre. Everyone is being so kind and I am stunned with how many people have been following my treatment journey. I decide I need to celebrate the day my book is launched, so I take myself out to lunch and celebrate alone. A time to reflect and eat chocolate fudge cake. Life is for living, after all.

KINDLY BLUNT INFORMATION

This is not my first book. Before my cancer story I wrote a book called "*I've Got Your Back – The Essential Guide to Marketing Your Therapy Business.*" Unlike a memoir, it's a practical business guide. My experience marketing this book and working as an expert for small business owners in online marketing gave me a head start when it came to selling *Agnes, Bea, Cancer and Me*. I already had a solid social media following. I had recruited an active advanced reader team who read the book ahead of time, offered feedback, and helped spread the word on launch day. On top of that, my business mentoring group, the HBClub, followed my cancer treatment journey closely and were eager to get their hands on a copy.

Rejected

Amidst all the positive feedback about the book was one irritating negative incident. Before I published my book, I had a dream that it would take pride of place in a local book shop in a village close to where I grew up. It was a small shop that regularly promoted local authors with events to celebrate them. I followed their guide on where the book had to be for them to purchase, I even dropped a copy off for them to see. My book is available on all the trade book sites where bookshops can order, but they still refused to have my book in the shop, stating it was "too much of a risk". I offered to drop off free copies that they could sell, keep the profit and reorder if they got sales, but they said no again. This hurt and still to this day when I see them promoting other local authors I wonder why they would not stock my book, especially with no risk to themselves. Sometimes things happen that push you forward and this is one of them. I spent 20 years of my life in that village and now only live 15 minutes away. I believe in small businesses supporting each other. I know from the talks I have given and from the multiple five star reviews of the book that it was more than good enough to sit on their shelves. The best bit is I can write about how they made me feel in this book, as we all know they will never stock it let alone read it.

TALKING ABOUT MY BOOBS

"I talk fast and wave my arms about"

I Have Funny Bones

My first book about my cancer journey, *Agnes, Bea, Cancer and Me*, has meant that I have been lucky enough to be invited to groups to do talks about my experience. I love being a speaker, whether I am speaking about the work I do or to share my cancer story. Just like my writing, I present as me, although in a book you have the luxury that you don't have to keep up, as I talk fast and wave my arms about.

The positive of this whole story has to be that I can help raise awareness of breast cancer and making sure people go for their routine testing. With my background as an osteopath, I can also share other pathology signs and symptoms when people should seek further testing. It is an honour to be able to share my story with others, and I hope I alert more people to get seen early when they suspect things are not normal in their health.

I have been told I have funny bones. However, in my training as an osteopath we never studied the bones that make you laugh. My talks are light-hearted, and although it's a story about a serious cancer diagnosis I tell it in such a way that people smile. Humour is my way of addressing a serious subject. It is how I got through my diagnosis and months of treatment. The best bit of most talks is when I pass around my prosthetic boobs for them all to see and feel. How many speakers get to show their boobs to the audience? In one such talk, I got my fake boobs out. As is the norm, I hand them to the front row of the audience to pass around the room. I picked a lady to take the Looky-Likey NHS boob and her face was a picture. She took the boob, her eyes squinting in horror, then immediately dropped it like it was a wild kitten I had put into her hand. "Yuck!" was her reaction as it fell with a splat to the floor, then it was picked up and passed around the room a bit like a hot potato with everyone trying to pass it on as quick as they could. The other fake boobs were not quite so shocking to the audience, as they don't look like a real boob. I knew at that moment I would be telling the tale in this book.

ONLY FOOLS AND HORSES

"Out the other side and able to celebrate life"

Peckham

One of the best things to come from this challenge thrown into my life is the drive to travel more and not delay visiting new places. Eddie has certainly embraced living life with me and as fellow cancer survivors we both know how fragile life is and how important it is to live it the best we can right now.

I have only been to Paris once. A trip away to sit on a board of European osteopaths looking at osteopathic standards. On that visit, I arrived at the Gare du Nord but found the taxi queue was going to take me forever. I was waved around the corner where, instead of more cars, I found the motorbike taxi rank. I have only been on a motorbike once and that was a scramble bike with three of us riding across a field. A scary moment from my youth, I would not want to repeat. The motorbike taxi had a mini armchair type setup, so I had no qualms in beating the car queue as I climbed on as pillion. I had a blanket cover on my knees and my hand luggage was strapped to the back. Fast-forward 20 minutes, and I am on the Paris roads in rush-hour traffic with a driver who is weaving in and out of the cars. I have a mic on my helmet so I could talk to the driver, but all he heard is me shrieking. My screams increased as he pulled in the wing mirrors to get through a gap as I imagined my knees about to get knocked off. I arrived at my destination exhilarated, scared witless but unscathed. When he asked if I would like him to pick me up for my return journey, I say yes without thinking. A memory made but it was really scary! I do not want to repeat this experience again, however.

Today this is my second trip to Paris, but as I have never experienced the city centre, Eddie has booked a bijou hotel opposite a cute boulangerie right in the middle of everything. We walk, we stop at cafes for bread, cheese, wine and visit all of the main sights. It is just the best trip and I can't believe, finally, I am out the other side and able to celebrate life again.

Eddie is on a roll with helping me live my life and soon a trip to New York is planned, another city I have never been to. New York is as brilliant and as crazy as I anticipated. We take a boat ride out to Liberty Island to get up close to the Statue of Liberty. It really is incredible. We see a show on Broadway after taking lunch at Ellen's Stardust Diner where the waiting staff sing as they serve. I wanted to step up and sing with them, but luckily I held myself back.

As we get on our flight home from New York, Eddie jokes that he needs to book Peckham as our next trip. I look at him blankly as I am not sure why he has chosen, randomly, Peckham in London. Then it dawns on me, as I see his smirk, that he is referring to "New York, Paris, Peckham", as written on the side of the Trotters' van in *Only Fools and Horses*. (Google it if you are too young to remember the UK TV comedy series.) I laugh out loud as I sit back into my seat and thank the universe for letting me live and for giving me the best husband. It is not long before I am asleep, dreaming of Del Boy and Rodney, and wondering what Peckham is really like. I will let you know.

HAIR

"I am old and I only have one boob"

I Lost My Personality

When I was going through chemotherapy, I remember how traumatised I was by losing my hair. There I was, having my life saved with chemotherapy, and I was focused on being upset about hair. Until you lose your hair you won't know how you will truly feel, but for me and the majority of people losing our hair is one of the worst things about this journey. Right or wrong, I felt like I lost my personality, my femininity and, on a practical level, the ability to bundle my hair up into a high ponytail. I mourned my hair.

I embraced a beanie hat instead of a wig as I thought a wig would be uncomfortable, and I knew I would be pulling it off during hot flushes. Also, what do you do with a wig when it's not on your head? I decided that losing my hair was short-term and, in my head, by getting a wig I was admitting it was going to be long-term. I do think if I lost my hair again that I would try a wig or, even better, a variety of wigs, but I am desperately hoping I will never have to go through it again. The realisation that handfuls of my beautiful hair were falling out was one of the worst days of my life.

I finished my chemotherapy on Christmas Eve and after a month or so "fluff" had appeared on my head. It reminded me of the fluff seen on young boys' chins just as they hit puberty. I was so worried that this was all the hair I would get back. It grew back more at the sides than on the top and for a while I looked like a rockhopper penguin. Not cool. Google a rockhopper to see what I mean. Of course, my hair didn't grow back as fast as I wanted it to. I was so impatient. I worried how it would grow back would it be the same or, as happens in some cases, a different texture and colour?

After a few months I had a covering of hair and of course my single chin hair was back and as thick and strong as ever. There should be some sort of deal with the chemo gods that when hair grows back it only comes back where you want it. Why can't you choose what hair does grow back when you have been through this sort of experience? I certainly would not have invited my chin hair back and, worse, a new one seems to have grown on the other side of my chin. I just need a third to create a plait.

My eyebrow hair filled in, but my eyelashes were slow to follow and I was anxious that they might not return. My nose hairs must have returned, although I did not specifically look for them, as my nose stopped dripping, when least expected, as it did during chemo. I looked like an Action Man toy with a number two haircut. My hair was still shorter than my husband's. I longed for a ponytail and as far as I was concerned this was painfully slow.

At the end of *Agnes, Bea, Cancer and Me*, I wrote about us having to delay our wedding celebrations to May after my "no sign of cancer" from the experts. I was desperate for my hair to grow for that day. I hoped for two inches by then, but it was not to be. I had a covering of hair that had come back light brown with a speckle of grey. I was frustrated, as I could not wear the tiara I had planned to wear as I just didn't have enough hair to make it stay on my head. I had bought my dress, shoes and tiara back in late 2019, before the Covid lockdown cancelled our original wedding date in May 2020, and then a year of cancer had followed to once again stop any hopes of celebrating our wedding. Originally I had planned an updo of highlighted blonde hair with the sparkling tiara. Instead, I felt I had rubbish hair that, no matter how hard I wished, would just not grow quickly enough. It didn't make me feel good, it felt boring, so in a rash moment I asked my hairdresser to bleach it white blonde. Full on peroxide, white. Safe to say, it was no longer boring. I finally wore my wedding dress with bleached blonde hair, one boob and an extra couple of stone in treatment weight squeezed into my beautiful dress. I have dreams of having those pictures redone one day. I have teared up just writing this, as it's still very emotional for me. I didn't want to look the way I did on my wedding celebration day, despite people telling me I looked great. Currently we don't have one picture of our wedding up in our house as I hate the reminder of how I looked.

My hair has continued to grow, and eight months after my last chemo session I had about two inches of hair and this is when the curls started to arrive. People warned me that it would likely return full of curls and they were not wrong. I have always had a wave in my hair, but this was ringlets. I felt like a cockapoo, or maybe more like a labradoodle, as I am 5ft 10in, so a larger curly-haired dog fits this story better. A couple of months on and it is longer, extremely curly and slightly out of control. Curls upon curls. Curls that for some reason insist on growing upwards. You try controlling upward curls. Everyone tells me they love it, but it's not what I want. I didn't ask for any of this, and I don't want this style of hair because it was not my choice. I know I should be grateful I am alive, but I want me back and I want it now.

People say flippantly, "Don't worry, it will grow back," and of course they are right, but to get it to shoulder length is going to take longer than I planned. It takes me until May 2023 and finally I can put my hair up in a mini, half-up half-down style ponytail. Oh, the joy of something so simple. For me it is a nod to the person I was before, although it is still many inches from my previous length.

I had many compliments when I was bald and I shall make sure I remind people regularly of my fine features, namely "shapely cheekbones", "chiselled jaw" and "great shaped head". I am surprised I didn't get modelling offers for head work based on these compliments. Instead, I think all that has happened is my head just got bigger. I also had many kind people who said they loved my hair short and I have to agree I did rock the short blonde look, and, my goodness, it takes seconds to style. The point, however, is that I didn't choose any of this and I am seriously angry it happened to me. I didn't choose to have cancer and I didn't want to lose my hair, a huge part of my identity. I am determined to get back as much of the old me as possible, and that means shoulder-length hair. It's a shame I don't have a button on my shoulder like my old Girl's World doll, whose hair grew when you pressed it, although it was only a clump from the middle of her head that grew.

A Wedding Celebration

Since I heard the brilliant news that my son was getting married, I have been on a mission to grow my hair and make sure I stay well enough for the day. I have put my children through enough stress and anxiety being sick and I feel so fortunate to have got through it so that I can attend. There was a point during treatment where there were no guarantees I would survive, and I shed many tears thinking I may not be around to see my adult children's weddings. I was so worried that at one point during treatment I asked my friend Jackie if she would stand in for me, if I didn't make it. I asked her to go with my daughter to choose a dress if I had passed away before the day. Not an easy conversation, but I wanted to know my Mother of the Bride role would be covered should the worst happen. But here I am, still in remission and with a head of beautiful hair. It is not quite back to my previous style, but good enough to have a "hairdo". So many people have asked me if I am going to wear a hat. My reaction is a full on, "No chance." I now have hair and I am going to show it off. I am determined to show everyone I am well and back to being Joe and Louise's mum rather than feeling like a burden.

I am about to be the Mother of the Groom, an important role, or at least I am telling myself it is. I need to look fabulous after months of squeezing into things with extra weight and longing for hair. I need a dress and not just any dress an outfit that befits the role of Mother of the Groom and, as is my "thing", shoes to die for (excuse the pun and perhaps inappropriate flippant mention of death in this book). I am one-boobed, with a prosthetic inserted into my bra, and larger than I used to be, so this is not going to be the easiest of missions. The dress needs to fit, I need to feel special in it and I am scared of anything with a V-neck now my cleavage area is now only a "vage" and not quite as it used to be. I decide I want to do this alone, perhaps to lessen the pressure of finding something, so I have booked myself a personal shopper in a large London department store and I am going on my own.

I arrive at the personal shopper area of Selfridges, where there are sofas and coffee tables. It seems very posh and suddenly I feel totally out of my comfort zone. I am also confused because there is no one around. I hang around for a bit and eventually ask a lady on another counter where I could find the personal shopper. She hurries off to find someone, but returns looking flustered and explains that they had not been told I was coming. They can see my appointment on the system, but no personal shopper had been allocated. My face must have dropped a mile, as she quickly adds that they will find someone and would I take a seat for a minute. I can see other members of staff flitting around and one in particular was a young man who obviously had very up-to-date fashion sense: cropped flared trousers and waistcoat ensemble. He looked fabulous, but in my head I was saying "Please not him, he is far too fashionable for someone like me." Of course, you can quickly guess who then walked over and introduced himself as my personal shopper. Yes, the very fashionable man I avidly did not want. I instantly felt sympathy for him having to find this old bird an outfit. He kindly asked what I was looking for. Instead of explaining like a normal person, I just blurted out, "I need a dress for my son's wedding, I am old and I only have one boob." This lovely man took my oversharing in his stride. He nodded and calmly said, "I am sure we can find you something, let's walk around the shop and you tell me what you like." Meanwhile I had the biggest hot flush, or was that a blush? I wonder how he will tell the same story this evening when he gets home.

Move on an hour and I have a beautiful dress that cost more than I have ever paid for an item of clothing, but it is perfect. As we walked around the store, the young salesman had suggested this dress among others but on the hanger it looked uninspiring. I was willing to try, although I had little confidence it would be *the* dress, but as soon as I put it on, I knew it was. It fitted perfectly and more importantly I felt fabulous. I have not felt fabulous in a long time and I am trying not to cry in front of my lovely helper. It has a variety of colours in the pattern with, in the main, dark pink and orange. I do try on other dresses, which despite eye-watering high price tags make me look terrible. I am obviously not made for designer looks or their price tags. Thankfully, I have my dress and I almost skip my way back to the tube clutching the posh dress bag with my valued prize inside. I have to share a huge thank you to the wonderful man who helped me feel great in the store. I apologise for judging him, please give that man a promotion and a wage rise. He dealt with the old girl with one boob with true professionalism.

Great Shoes

I love shoes, so the next job is to get some great shoes. Throughout my life I have always placed a lot of importance and money on fabulous shoes. The shoes, however, are not as easy to find as the dress, but the universe seems to have ideas to help my choice. I spent a few days out shopping, but I can't find suitable shoes that I love. I have seen a pair of ombre pink and orange shoes on a website, but I felt the heels were too high and, even for me who loves shoes, way too expensive, so I held back from purchasing them.

As part of my living life, we have planned 10 days away in Fuerteventura, and whilst I am sitting by the pool checking my phone I notice an email to say the same shoes are now in the sale. Now, I really am interested in them, but I am away so I can't order them as the parcel would have to sit on the doorstep for another week. I will have to wait until I get home and hope they are still available in my size when I return. We get home 10 days later and, to my relief, the sale is still on and they have a pair in my size. But the story gets better, I told you the universe was looking out for me on the shoes. I was blown away to receive an email saying they wanted to offer more money off and 20 percent of the sale would be donated to Cancer Research. A total coincidence. Talk about a pair of shoes that were meant to be mine. Soon the shoes arrive and I am in love with them. They are high, but I have sat in them, walked in them to stretch the leather and, as far as high-heeled stilettos can be, they are comfortable. Anyone that has worn heels knows that I am using the word "comfortable" very loosely.

Fingers Up To Cancer Today

What a fabulous day today. It is my son's wedding. A day to celebrate and welcome my daughter-in-law, into the family. Today feels like a new start, a day I wasn't sure I would see, but here I am at the hairdressers getting my hair and makeup done before setting off to the venue. It's fun in my house today. My son and the groomsmen are getting ready there. The buzz at home is electric, although I am glad I have popped out to have a little peace, whilst being made beautiful, before heading back to them all. Time to reflect on how fortunate I am to have got through a serious cancer diagnosis and how grateful I am to be allowed to be part of this day.

We get to the venue and I feel great, a feeling that has been eluding me for what seems years. I feel like Mum again, rather than Helen who had cancer. My hair has been done and, although it is not quite as long I would want it, it is a real style and it looks nice. I have my beautiful dress on and killer heels. I chose to not have a hat as I want to show my hair off now that I have it again.

I love my shoes. I love them so much that as I sit in my "Mother of the Groom, I am very important" aisle seat, I make sure I cross my legs so that one of my beautiful shoes sticks out for all to see. I make myself giggle at my shoe show and I promise I only did this before the bride walked down the aisle. I may not have two boobs, but the prosthetic I have chosen to wear is doing a good job to create symmetry. I look and feel bloody awesome. I have so many lovely comments about my hair, dress and shoes, and I manage to keep the shoes on until 8pm when the dancing starts, at which point I slip into a pair of comfy trainers to dance the night away. Everyone comments how well I look, and today I feel it too. Life is good and I am truly thankful I am alive to make their celebrations without causing them any worry. This is definitely a fingers up to cancer type of day. I am on the dance floor enjoying the bright disco lights and I have not felt the dark shadow all day.

KINDLY BLUNT REMINDER

You are more than your external appearance. I valued my hair and it hurt so much losing it, but look at me today. Alive, dancing and smiling the broadest smile. I must insist that everyone needs nice shoes – your personality is not lost when you have cancer. Deep inside you are still there, perhaps a little broken, but your essence is still there and those that love you are waiting for you to shine again. Smile hard and watch those around you smile back.

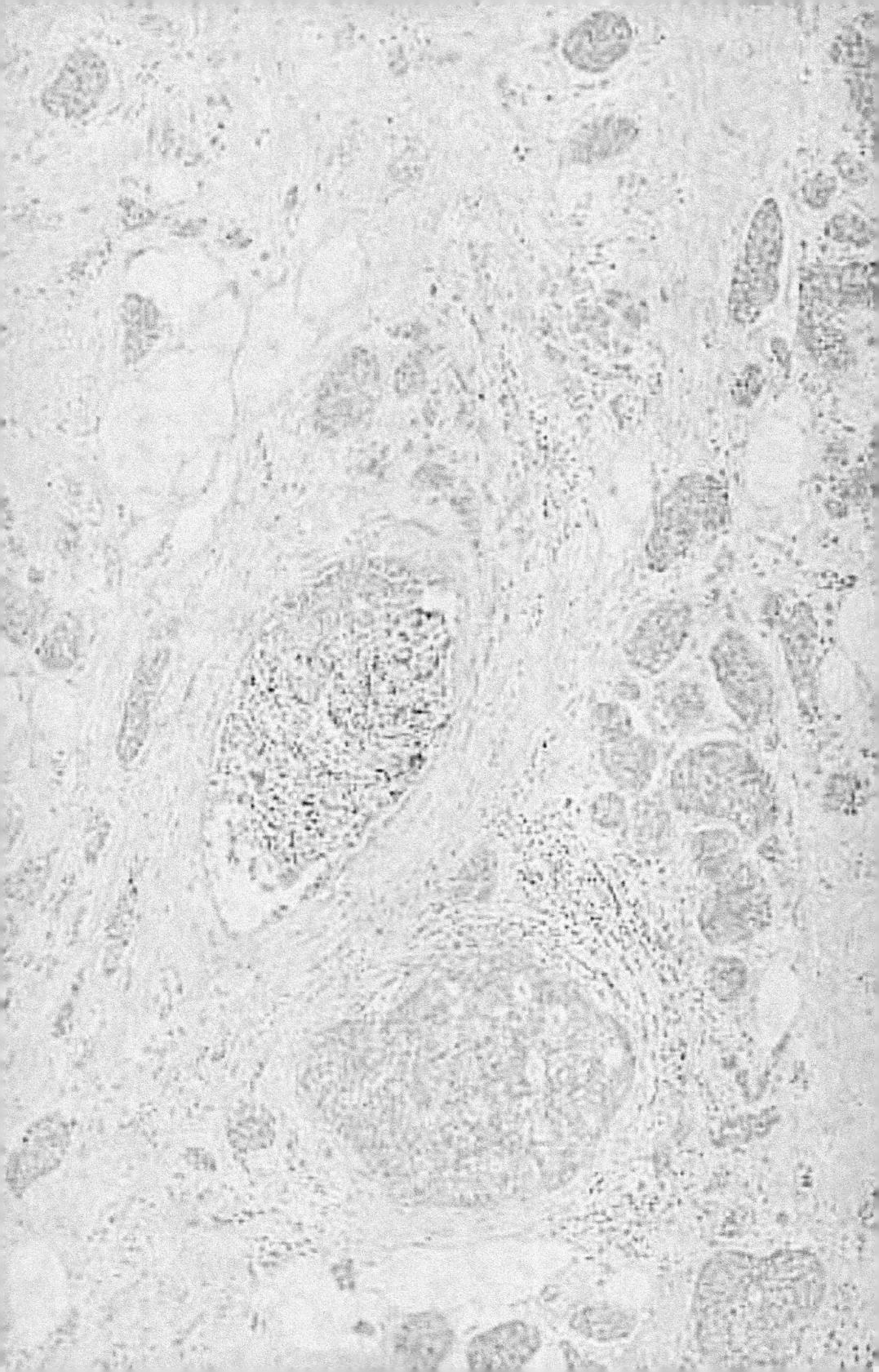

Decisions To Be Made

A DILEMMA

"So many what if's are passing through my brain"

I Miss My Clea

Time seems to have gone fast, but it feels like a lifetime since I had two boobs. Way back in 2021, I had a cleavage. Two boobs called Agnes and Bea. Agnes was the "clea" to Bea's "vage", but now all I am left with is Bea. You may be wondering why I miss having a whole cleavage. With one boob it is hard to have symmetry in clothes. Of course, I can wear a prosthetic boob to create the illusion of symmetry, but I find it annoying and uncomfortable. The second reason is when I do exercise. A prosthetic boob is not practical. As an example, today I went for a run, or, more accurately, a waddling type of shuffle with a small amount of forward momentum. It was still dark outside, so I put on a cross-body running light that I wear when I go out in the winter months. I am struggling to see as I shuffle along, because the light keeps veering off to the right. No matter how much I tighten the straps and readjust the light, it keeps moving. This is strange, as it has never happened before. Then it dawns on me. I now only have a "vage". My chest light, ironically named in this case, has nothing to anchor itself on and is being pushed across to my right by Bea. I chuckle to myself as I hold the light in place and finish my run. Who knew having only one boob would affect my running too?

My World Is Turned Upside Down

Just before my son's wedding day, I made the decision that I would get the reconstruction surgery. Quite a surprise, as it took me such a long time to decide, but as I had remained in the system I was already on the surgery pathway unless I had decided to pull the plug. I asked the medical team if I could be called after October 2023 as I didn't want to be recovering from major surgery at my son's wedding. My kids have seen me sick too much for my liking and I wanted to be fit, well and able to dance the night away at his wedding. The wedding is over, so now it's a waiting game for the date to come through. I have asked the team and it looks like I have to wait until next year. I am keen to get on with things, but of course I have to wait my turn.

Today is a fun day, as it is the time of year when I get together with my friends to plan our annual pre-Christmas week away. There are 10 of us, who for more years than I can remember have been going away every November. I think it is around 20 years since we started doing this, but I have to confess it could be even longer. I jump on my bike and cycle to my friend's house for a coffee and a chat about things we need to do before we go. We have been away together for so many years that we pretty much know what we need. We have rented a house and now it's time to organise the food shop.

I am really looking forward to getting away this year, as I almost feel like me again and I am ready to do all the normal things I used to do before cancer. We sit discussing the weekend and allocating jobs to each person. Just as I volunteer to make cakes for the weekend, my phone rings. I can see it is the hospital number so I excuse myself and answer the call. Suddenly my world is turned upside down. It is the hospital secretary letting me know they have had a cancellation and I am being offered the slot, but it is in just

10 days' time. The exact same day I should be leaving for the girls' weekend. The secretary on the phone has more details for me to digest. If I want the surgery and to not wait until an unknown time next year, this operation will be done by a different surgeon. I take a deep breath of excitement and anxiety as I wonder why nothing is simple on this shit journey. I want surgery as soon as I can, but I don't know this new surgeon and I won't get to meet them until I am being prepped for the operation if I take this surgical slot. I get off the call and apologise to my friends that I will have to go home, as I really can't focus on much else right now. The secretary needs an answer from me in an hour. I am soon back on my bicycle, hurriedly cycling home to discuss it all with Eddie.

I have a dilemma. I want the operation as soon as possible, as it would mean surgery would be done by Christmas, with family around me as I recover. I will be fully recovered by my daughter's wedding in August next year. But I am nervous about seeing another surgeon, a surgeon I won't meet until the day of my operation. A lady surgeon was originally assigned to me. I have met her twice and I liked her. I have no real idea of how good she would be, but I had confidently put my trust in her. Now I have an hour to ring back the secretary to claim the slot or lose it to the person next on the waiting list. I open up my PC and do the best research I can on Google in the short amount of time I have. I put the new surgeon's name into Google and to my relief his credentials are not just good, they are excellent. He qualified in medicine from Oxford University, during his masters in surgical science he got the highest distinction in his year, he was given an award for his work and he specialises in breast reconstruction. As I read, it just gets better and better. I am imagining my newly allocated plastic surgeon as a superhero with great sewing skills. I can't, however, find any evidence that he is good at dressmaking or that he owns a superhero cape.

Now I need to act fast. I double check with Eddie that he is onboard with me taking this opportunity. Then I grab my phone, call the consultant's secretary and accept the appointment. I will have to miss this years girls' weekend, but it is for good reason. My operation date is set for 22nd November. I am excited and scared witless in equal amounts. So many what if's are passing through my brain. Should I have such serious surgery? Am I risking too much? Will this go to plan? More seriously, do I have a pair of pyjamas that is good enough to take to hospital?

Polo-Neck Knickers

Over the next week, I am on high alert and it is a real rush to try to get ready for my operation. I have a list of things they have asked me to take in, and that includes two special post-surgery bras and big pants. When I say big pants, I am talking the biggest and tightest pants I have ever seen. They go right up to my bust line. I call them "polo-neck knickers" as they come up so high. Most women will have worn control pants at some point in their lives, and they will know how uncomfortable they are. Getting home from a party and removing them is a priority. I am going to have to wear these for at least six weeks, day and night, to control the swelling. These pants may be big, but conversely they are also small when you try to pull them up. Tight would be an understatement. I am now the proud owner of six pairs of polo-neck knickers. I wanted to buy all black, but there were only four black and two beige-coloured on the shelf. I have decided that no one should ever wear beige-coloured pants. It is not a good look and I laugh inwardly as I show Eddie my passion-killer polo-neck knickers. He tries to hide his shock and horror, without success.

I am excited and nervous to finally be having my reconstruction operation, but it is also tinged with sadness that I am missing out on the fun of the girls' weekend. I don't trust yet that cancer won't return and with that I have no certainty that I will be alive next year to go away with them all. This may sound dramatic, but the feelings are real. I have mixed emotions as I pack my bag for the operation ahead.

KINDLY BLUNT OBSERVATION

Never wear beige-coloured pants. I am sure they are as bad for your health as a beige buffet. Go for glorious colours in your underwear drawer. If nothing else, it will make you smile. Beige will never make you or anyone around you happy.

BUILD A BOOB

"If you have never worn paper pants..."

Sewing Bea

Finally, 20 months since Agnes was taken from me during a right-sided mastectomy, it is the day of my DIEP reconstruction. I am elated and terrified at the same time. I wonder if there is a point that you experience so many emotions in such a short time that you implode? I feel I may implode today. My head is a mess. There have been many times during my cancer journey that I wonder how I got myself into so much trouble. This is a journey I could have never imagined that I would go through, and I am still in shock that it happened to me.

I made my final decision to have the reconstruction after seeing the plastic surgeon and learning about my belly transplant and all the little extras they would do at the same time. Although this is a big draw, the real reason is that I am fed up wearing a false boob, as it is just a faff to find it, put it in place and try to remain comfortable for long periods of time. I am bored with it all and I want a symmetrical shape to add back a "clea" to my "vage". I want to be able to buy bras that fit easily. More than that, I want to buy pretty bras without thoughts of "will the false boob fit?" I want to pull on a top and not worry whether the front is too low or that my prosthesis will move, get hot, feel heavy or look odd. I admit, I am lazy when it comes to my appearance. I like to look nice, but

I certainly do not want it to take too much effort. Wearing a fake boob for the last 20 months now feels like effort.

Today we are on our way to the specialist plastic surgery hospital for my "Build a Boob" operation. I suspect it is going to be nothing like those "Build a Bear" shops where you choose a bear and watch it get stuffed before your eyes. As always, Eddie is at the wheel, making sure I get there on time. I am not sure I would be fit to drive as I am so anxious my hands are shaking. As with all operations, I have not eaten for many hours. Instead, I did have to endure the disgusting carbohydrate drinks last night and first thing this morning. I am not good with a milkshake so giving me multiple bottles of gloopy drink is never going to be a pretty picture. Of course, I drank them, but not without a lot of moaning and retching. Eddie honestly deserves an award with the amount he has had to put up with.

This DIEP operation is classed as major surgery and will take at least eight hours to complete with more than one surgeon working on me. I have visions of it being like the TV programme *The Great British Sewing Bee*, with the surgeons as the contestants being given their second-hand garment that they have to recycle and create something amazing from. It really will be a Sewing of Bea, as she is about to get a surgical lift as one of my DIEP surgery bonuses.

We arrive at the waiting room way before normal people have their breakfast. Poor Eddie normally would not be out of bed yet, but he is putting on a brave face and I know he is tired and worried too. Together we sit outside the surgery waiting room, my bag in hand, which is full of PJs, massive pants and the most supportive, deep bras you can imagine. I am understandably nervous of both the surgery and the huge underwear. This surgery is going to take me a minimum of 12 weeks to recover from. Just as I wonder if I am making the right decision putting myself through more surgery, the door to the waiting room is opened and I am waved in. Eddie jumps up to join me but it seems I have to do this part alone as the nurse shakes her head. I say my goodbyes to Eddie at the door, trying not to cry, pretending I am brave, and walk through to another world that I have been forced to be part of. I am asked to take a seat and I spend my time watching people saying goodbye to loved ones at the door whilst straining to hold back my tears.

It is not long before I am called through to an examination room. Blue NHS disposable curtains drawn around an area is something that has become part of my new normal. The nurse does all the health checks necessary before any operation, then asks me to undress, put on the obligatory gown that flaps open at the back, the most attractive green surgical stockings and paper pants. If you have never worn paper pants, you are one lucky person. I don't know who designed them, but they have no shape. Perhaps it is hard to shape paper and elastic, but they are certainly not designed for comfort like my faithful M&S pants. I think they got two squares of paper towel, stitched across the bottom and part way down the side leaving a hole for my legs and then dropped some cheap elastic around the top and leg holes. Mine are slightly tighter than I would wish for. I would say I feel like I have lost my dignity, but that went months ago.

My anxiety increases as I sit and await the arrival of the surgeon, a man I have never met due to the last-minute swap. Thankfully, it is not long before he arrives with another surgeon, who I assume is still in training for this type of operation. The second surgeon is very knowledgeable, but looks to the lead surgeon for advice. I am asked to undress, and I can't tell you how awful it feels to be standing in front of two men and a female nurse chaperone in my paper pants and surgical stockings. Of course, there is no other way this can be done, and I have learnt to remove myself mentally from all the uncomfortable situations I have been put through over the last few years. Today I choose to look straight ahead and thank my lucky stars there is no mirror. I should also apologise to you as it's likely you now have a vision of me in your head, which I know is not pretty.

Meat In The Butcher Shop

I was always told measure twice, cut once and that is how it feels they are working as they get a Sharpie and mark up my body. Measurements are made to check the lengths of my clavicles, my ribcage and many other reference points for when I am in surgery. Bea is lifted manually by the surgeon to assess her new potential position. I do hope she is happy getting an uplift during all of this. My mastectomy scar, where Agnes used to be, will be opened up and the fat from my abdomen will form my new boob shape. I can't help but laugh out loud when the surgeon congratulates me on my fabulous abdominal blood vessels. He goes on to tell me that from my scan they look like they are perfectly sized. This, he tells me, will increase the chances of the operation being a success when they plumb my tummy tissue blood vessels to my chest blood vessels. As usual, I can't help but say something random, so I tell him all about me having the perfect head shape and jaw line when I was bald. I was trying to tell him I had many surprisingly good body parts. This is certainly one of my distraction attempts, but I am not sure he needed to hear it. He is kind enough to smile at me, slightly confused, and then get straight back to his work colouring in my body with his Sharpie pen. I shall, however, be telling everyone about my perfect body parts whenever I can after all of this.

My mind is doing somersaults as I try to look nonchalant with all the chat between the surgeons about my body. It really is an out of body experience hearing them talk about me in this way. Of course, they are professional and I respect that, but it is hard not to feel like a piece of meat in the butcher shop. Next, another surgeon is introduced to me who will also be part of the team. I am surprised to learn that three surgeons will be working on me during this reconstruction and the reality of this being major surgery hits me hard. I stare straight ahead and try to imagine this is not happening to me. It is surreal and, despite their best efforts to be kind, informative and preserve my modesty, there really is no way to mark me up for reconstruction surgery without me feeling embarrassed. I will never be able to look at a Sharpie again in the same way. I imagine I look like a child who has found a felt tip and had fun drawing all over themselves. At least they didn't have to write "This Way Up" anywhere.

Finally the surgical team are finished and happy that I am covered in a join-the-dots type of pattern for the reconstruction. The nurse then gives me the pre-med drugs and I start to feel a little drowsy. I seem to be an expert in general anaesthetic these days and I note that, unusually, I walk myself down to the operating theatre instead of being on a trolley. When I had Agnes removed I was wheeled down to theatre, put in a little bay just outside and put to sleep there. This time I walk myself down the corridor and straight into the operating theatre. The room is full of bright lights, which of course is good for threading needles and sewing things neatly, but quite scary to walk into. I am, however, happy that the room looks tidy and sterile. Of course, it needs to be like this, but in my head I hate clutter and I equate tidy to neat work being done here. All good so far.

I climb up onto the operating table, the bright lights making me squint. Now I am scared and all my bravado and joking has disappeared. Seeing my anxiety, the anaesthetist calmly holds my arm and says, "Hi, we have got you." I don't know why, but I appreciate the informal greeting from this doctor. He is really nice and explains what is going on and that he will be working with another anaesthetist. He jokes that someone needs to be there when he eats his ham sandwich. It is the first time it dawns on me that this team will need breaks. Eight hours is a long time and they will need food breaks, toilet breaks and I assume time off during this huge operation. He explains there is also a physiotherapist who will come in part of the way through to move my limbs around, as I will be lying flat for so long, not that I am going to know anything about it. I have no idea how many are in the team, but so far I count at least six of them and that does not include the nurses. The team work to carefully position me so that they can access all areas. This *Great British Sewing Bee* challenge of making old into new is really going to be tough for them today. Just as I start to worry that they have an impossible task ahead of them, I am given the anaesthetic. I start to count back..., 10, nine and I am asleep. I have the easiest part in this operation. I am asleep and time will pass by fast, but I have a team that will be working all day on me, and Eddie is at home having to wait and worry for hours before receiving any news.

In total my operation takes eight and a half hours, not that I have any awareness of that. In my head I was counting back from 10 and then almost instantly someone was asking me to wake up. I remember smiling as I woke, feeling I had just had the best deep sleep. It was also relief that I felt no pain, unlike waking after my mastectomy operation, when for a few minutes I was in excruciating pain before they pumped me full of morphine. I remember as I was coming in and out of consciousness that I was saying thank you to everyone. I have no idea who anyone was as I was still heavily medicated, but I do remember the porter laughing as I said thank you to everyone we passed as he pushed me down corridors to the ward. He reported to the nurses on my arrival that I thanked many people we passed who were nothing to do with my operation, including hospital visitors and he shared with the nursing staff that he liked how polite I was.

After seemingly thanking everyone in the hospital, I finally arrive on a ward with four beds. One bed is empty and the others are already filled with two other ladies who have had a similar operation. I find it amazing that three surgical teams have been working on us all most of the day. During the operation they have put me into one of my front-loading big bras, required after this type of surgery. I am hardly awake and already the checks are starting. I was warned that I would be checked hourly straight after surgery to check that the blood supply was flowing at the surgery site. I am confident that my fabulous blood vessels are going to work well. The nursing team use a doppler ultrasound to check the blood flow. I was warned during the show-and-tell session that I went to that the doctors call the site of the new belly boob a "flap". Despite being still woozy with the meds it makes me smile that the doctors keep asking to see my "flap"! I make a mental note not to show them the wrong part of my body.

Thankfully, I can hear the whooshing of the blood as they use the doppler over the transferred tissue and the nurse cleverly marks the best spot for hearing it on my new boob. Another Sharpie mark on my body. This means the next person that checks can find the place easily. I have a blood pressure cuff on my arm that at regular intervals inflates, and I have inflatable sleeves that go up and down on my legs to help blood circulate and prevent blood clots. I am given a button in my hand to administer strong medication if I need it, and the nurse tells me to use it before the pain gets too bad. I have to press the button many times during the night as I don't want it to hurt. They did tell me I would be checked regularly but I had not realised there would be no time to sleep, with nurses at my side making their checks all through the night. So many checks, including blood pressure, blood flow to the new flap and even blood-thinning injections being given as I drift in and out of sleep. It was a long night of interruptions but of course it had to be done.

As I lie trying to sleep between all the checks, I count up the scars I now have after the operation. In total I have seven scars. My stomach scar runs from hip to hip, Bea has three scars from her uplift and the new belly boob has two. Then there's my belly button scar, which, because they remove the excess flesh from the stomach area and pull the remaining tissue down to join things up, shows they have moved my belly button. If they left my belly button untouched it would be very low, so instead they popped it up through a bit of skin higher up. I have no idea what any of it looks like right now as it is all covered, but I am keeping my fingers crossed. The thought of stitches makes me feel sick, whether they are on me or anyone else. I guess you would call me squeamish and even thinking about it makes me squirm. I am very glad they are all currently under heavy bandages. I could write loads about how uncomfortable I am, but I think with seven scars after an eight-hour operation that would be no surprise and you can fully imagine how I feel right now.

I am to stay in hospital for a few more days, so Eddie, my daughter Louise and my lovely friend Jackie (Jackie has her own chapter in my previous book) come and visit me. The nurses are great and the next day I am helped to standing and into the chair beside my bed. I can't believe how difficult it is to move. It could just be the large, tight-fitting underwear, but of course I know it is more than that. I feel like they have sewn everything together too tight as I am bent double when I move. I seriously wonder if I have made a mistake in getting this done.

Oh Poop

Today the medical team have started to talk about letting me go home, but first I have to be able to walk to the toilet unaided. I have just had the catheter taken out and the medical team are anxious I have my first pee. Going to the toilet is a simple task, you may think, but I am attached to two drains and I can't stand upright. Walking a few metres to the toilet seems like an impossible task and the first time I try I feel faint, so I am told to wait a while. Finally, I manage to get the strength to get to the toilet, but then I just can't pee, it's like I have forgotten how to. The nurses are anxious I keep trying, so I decide to do some laps of the corridor to get things moving. Laps of the corridor is an exaggeration instead I walk 10 slow paces forward and then I turn around carefully and go back, as that is all that I can manage. After quite some time and after way longer than any of the other women on my ward, I finally manage to pee. Celebrations are had all around as everyone is aware of my predicament. Next it is time to see if my drains can come out. I am adamant I do not want to come home with drains attached to me. I was sent home with drains after my mastectomy and I hated it. Back then, having a mastectomy and being sent home the same day was a serious shock to my system. This time it is different, as I have been in hospital for a few days; to my relief the drains are removed. The removal of drains is not the nicest thing to have done, but better than taking them home attached to me. Now I only have one hurdle left to get over to get home. I need to open my bowels, or in layman's terms, do a poo. I need to pass a stool before I am able to go home, but try having major abdominal surgery, a load of constipation-making meds and then producing a poo. In my case it is impossible. Is this going be what holds me back from leaving? In my usual fashion, I manage to talk my way out of having to stay any longer. I promise the team that I will be able to pass a stool at home, and I am not sure exactly how I will do it, but I convince them I can go home. I rush to call Eddie and get the hell out of there. No disrespect to the care I have received; I just want to get home.

A few hours later, Eddie has arrived and helps me gather all my things together. The next hurdle is to get out of the hospital. I slowly shuffle along the long corridor to the car park with many rests along the way. Everything seems difficult, but I have been cut about and remodelled so it's hardly surprising. Getting into a low car and then working out how to twist my legs into the footwell is another hurdle. Then comes the seatbelt. Where do you put a seatbelt when you have had surgery over most of the front of your body at all the points a seatbelt sits? I have two cushions that I stuff into place behind the belt, but I am dreading the journey home like this. The previously simple drive seems like a lifetime and I am glad to get home, as it proves a very painful journey.

I arrive home with a bag of bandages, surgical tape, painkillers and, of course, my bag full of large polo-neck knickers. If you have ever worn support pants for a few hours you know the relief when you take them off, but I am not allowed to go without them for at least six weeks. Night and day I have to wear the big pant passion-killers. Not that passion is an area I will be thinking about for a while. The compression bra is the same, supportive but uncomfortable when worn 24 hours a day. Oh, and don't forget the knee-high support stockings to help prevent blood clots. If it wasn't so uncomfortable it would be funny!

I get home and I am in post-operation shock. I have been running on adrenalin for the last few days and now the reality of this massive operation sinks in. The discomfort is real and, with so many large scar sites, I am in a lot of pain. I have been instructed to sleep on my back in a semi-recumbent position, but for a usual side sleeper I am finding it impossible to sleep more than about 30 mins. After lying awake most of the night, I decide to go downstairs and try our recliner sofa, and for the next four weeks I spend the night under my duvet on the sofa. I still can't sleep for more than a few hours before waking as I am very uncomfortable. It's lonely at 3am as everyone else sleeps.

I Have Made A Mistake

I am starting to think I have made a mistake with this operation. Almost five weeks have passed and the lack of sleep, discomfort and tight underwear is driving me mad. My wounds need dressing almost daily and it takes time with so many surgical sites. Stitches have always made me feel sick and after five weeks that feeling has not gone away. But here I am with the surgery done and I have to dig deep and just get on with it. I didn't think this was going to be so hard. Was this the right decision?

Today I am back to the hospital for my post-six-week check. I still have tape on my wounds, but I am feeling a little better in myself. I am almost able to walk totally upright, even if I am still slow. The specialist nurse takes a look at my wounds and to my delight tells me the dressings can come off and I can stop wearing such supportive underwear. I am ecstatic to no longer have to wear such restrictive undergarments. I share with her that looking at or touching my new belly button makes me feel sick. She reassures me most women feel like this and tells me to touch it while she is there. My new belly button position is higher than it used to be and I feel queasy as I touch it. I don't have proper feeling over my abdomen and it just feels odd. Once I have touched it she then tells me to stick my finger in it. Yuk, why does it make me feel nauseous? I do it and of course it is not as bad as I thought, although I won't be doing it again soon. The good news today is that they are happy all the surgical sites have healed and, apart from still not lifting anything or any overexertion for another six weeks, I am allowed to go home tape free. If I could, I would be skipping out of there!

A couple of weeks after seeing the nurse it's a joy not having to redress wounds every few days. It is also a treat to be able to get into the shower and stay under the water without worrying the bandages need changing or drying afterwards. Today, however, I notice that one area of the wound on the new belly boob looks like it is opening up. If I said I was a bit hysterical about my wounds, I would be under selling it. I am so anxious that it all heals well, and my head quickly goes into overdrive when I see this wound is not healing properly. I am straight on the phone to the medical team. They are fast to respond and recommend I use silver bandages over the wound to help healing. The next day the silver products arrive in the post and for the next week I have to bathe the wound daily in saltwater and cover with the silver dressings. Unfortunately, there is no improvement; instead, the next time I get into the shower with the dressing off there is blood and pus everywhere. I look down and see that the wound opening is even bigger and the water of the shower is making it look 10 times worse. The area is now about the size of a five-pence piece and there is no mistaking the wound has opened and is getting worse.

I phone the nursing team and they call me in right away to see the medical team. Almost immediately they diagnose a stitch abscess. They explain this is where my wound has hyper-granulation which is stopping the stitches from dissolving and the wound from healing. Granulation is the normal healing process, but my body has done things to the extreme. Extreme is typical of me in most things in my life. My biggest worry is that I am due to be on holiday in two weeks, and if the wound does not heal I will not be able to enter the water. In our living life theme we have booked a trip to Barbados and Antigua, and I am really anxious and angry that this is going to spoil things. The nurse is kind and empathises with my frustration that only a few weeks ago I was given the go-ahead to relax as the wounds seemed healed. She cauterizes the wound and with some extra care it should heal. It is touch and go as to whether I can go swimming in two weeks but, I have another appointment with my plastic surgeon the day before we go away so I am hopeful. The nurse is not confident that it will be healed in time, but I have my fingers crossed.

Fingers Crossed

Today I am back to the hospital for my 12-week check with the surgeon. We are packed and ready to fly to the Caribbean tomorrow and I am still keeping my fingers crossed that I will be told I can go swimming while we are away. The surgeon seems pleased with my results and he gives the good news that my wound is almost healed, and if I use waterproof plasters for the first few days, I can go swimming on my holiday. I am also given the go-ahead to go back to normal life. I can lift, carry and workout without having to be careful. This news is the best I have had for a long while and we travel home looking forward to the most amazing holiday. I like my new body and it is time to make the most of life again! What better way to celebrate than on a white beach?

A Real Boob

When I first thought about having DIEP reconstruction surgery I worried that moving belly fat to my chest area would look odd. I imagined it looking as if a lump of my body was just stuck onto another area. I really thought it would look strange, but in reality, I now have a shape that looks like a real boob where Agnes once sat. It doesn't look like it was just stuck on. It truly is a fantastic feat of surgery and I am so thankful, now the worst is over, that I had it done. It was a long journey but now I have my cleavage back and symmetry. I feel great and look forward to wearing bikinis and V-neck tops again.

FABULOUS HOLIDAY

"I am embracing my new body"

In A Pickle

I am on yet another great holiday. Living my life to the full is fun and I am so grateful that we are able to experience so many nice things after such a tough time. I am, however, aware how fortunate I am. At last, I no longer feel that I am in a boxing ring having to put up a fight. The constant high alert of going through treatment and operations is subsiding and today I feel hopeful. I can't remember the last time I was truly hopeful in this whole journey and it feels great.

We have just arrived at the most glorious hotel in Barbados, our home for 10 days before we then jet off to Antigua for the second half of our holiday. I should be pinching myself to check this is real. My wound is healing and I am going to try swimming tomorrow, as my surgeon has given me the go-ahead. Gratitude is high on my list today. I notice as I sit by the pool in a bikini with two boobs and a flat tummy that I no longer feel different from everyone else around me. Of course, I could wish to be younger, lighter, with less weight on my thighs, but all in all I am back to feeling like me again. I no longer feel like a cancer patient with a check-up appointment always just around the corner. I was diagnosed in the second half of 2021 and finally in January 2024 I no longer feel different. It has been a long road to this feeling, but finally I think I am turning a huge corner.

I am only just 12 weeks post surgery so I still have to be conscious I don't overstretch myself; however, my body is good at telling me as physically I can't overdo it. It's day two of our holiday and finally I can get in the pool. Swimming, however, is surprisingly difficult. Trying to do breaststroke with arms and legs moving in opposite directions is uncomfortable with a new abdomen that is now very tight. I set myself some rehab exercises to do in the pool as I am determined to regain all my range of movement back. It's fortunate I am a retired osteopath as rehab exercises are simple for me to create and water is the perfect medium to rebuild my strength.

After over a week in Barbados I am so chilled. We have a hotel that has a restaurant right on the edge of the beach, with amazing food each day. I am enjoying the slow pace and as each day passes I am less and less conscious of my scars. My swimming rehab is going well, and daily I have walked along the white sands to increase my stamina. After 10 wonderful days we are now off to see another island. Today we are off to Antigua.

Frustratingly, we arrive on this beautiful island in the rain after leaving glorious sun in Barbados, but as we reach our villa looking over the water, the sun returns. I can't believe we have another 10 days away from all the worry and stress, and every day I feel stronger. My body is healing and with that comes a return of more movement. In fact, I am feeling so much better that today we are off to try out pickleball. I have never played it before, but I am told it is like mini tennis. I am right-handed and I obviously have a lot of scars healing on that side. However the consultant has told me I can go back to doing anything I want, so I am determined to give it a go. We head on down to join the hotel-organised group session but when we get there everyone else seems to be an expert in the game. I can only describe it as being like tennis but with a smaller court, plastic ball and different rules about areas of the court and when you can volley the ball. Oddly, part of the court is called the "kitchen". The paddle racquet is solid and the ball is plastic with holes in it. The group we have joined are American and all know each other. They tell us they have travelled specifically to this hotel for the pickleball courts. As this is an open session for all they greet us enthusiastically and show us how to play. Eddie and I pair up and give it a go. I choose the left side so Eddie can cover me from stretching too far to the right and we start to play. Both Eddie and I have good hand-eye co-ordination, so hitting a ball is easy for us. I am also a volleyball player who in my younger years played in the top league in the UK and that is helping too. Before we know it, we have won all three games against the people that taught us. We don't seem so popular now we have beaten seasoned players, so we quietly say thank you and slope off, secretly laughing at our audacity as we go. We did have a few cocktails at the bar to celebrate.

Blissful days are passing as we chill out by the pool and the beach. I am so relaxed and perhaps because the sun is so bright, I have not once thought of the dark shadow of cancer while we have been away. It's a blessing and a relief.

Our hotel has a sister hotel and today we head off in a chauffeured golf buggy to the beach next door. Eddie is quick to notice a volleyball court by some of the sunbeds and, at week 14, post my operation, I find myself on a beach volleyball court holding my own with other players. Of course I can't play as I used to, due to operation restrictions and my age, but I explain to those around me that I won't be diving or hitting hard and I stick to those rules just to be safe. Another tick on the list of getting back to doing normal things again. I have a way to go before I am not worrying that I may split my scars open, but in reality that is very unlikely to happen.

Rum!

Today we are on a boat trip. I have been in the pool and the sea every day to try to increase my strength when swimming, and I feel ready to snorkel off the boat. It's hard going as we swim a long way out and back again, following a guide showing us all the key areas of the reef, but although I am exhausted when we finally get back on the boat, I do manage it. It is only 14 weeks since my operation and I could never have imagined how far I have come since those first days of struggling to walk a few steps. It has felt like a lifetime, but has also been an amazing recovery.

After our snorkel adventure, Eddie and I sip rum and enjoy the boat ride with music and dancing. Eddie enjoys far more rum than me and is very "happy" by the time we get off the boat. On returning to our hotel, as has become our norm, we go via the crazy-golf course on the way back up the hill to our villa. Others on our tour jump in the chauffeured golf buggies back to their villas, but we choose to walk as I am trying to increase my fitness. Today, fuelled by a lot of rum, we take on the crazy-golf course. I think you may be able to imagine how we get on, so there is no need for much description, but I will say we belly laughed all the way around, hit balls into the water obstacles and lost a few balls out of bounds. A belly laugh is something I have missed over the last few years, and despite the slight discomfort it feels good. Today I really feel like I am living the best life.

Finally, it is time to fly home from our adventure. This has been the perfect last piece of my post-operation recovery. I am embracing my new body despite the upsurge of emotions as I return to my reality of constant checks with the hospital. Almost as soon as the plane lands, I can feel that shadow returning. We arrive home to a pile of post, most of which are letters with more medical appointments to attend.

Bubbling Under The Surface

Post-cancer, I assumed I would always feel happy as being cancer free was all I thought of during my treatment. But the reality is the fear of cancer returning is always in the back of my mind. We have been back from holiday five days and today I have woken up with a rash on Bea. My first knee-jerk reaction is that I now have cancer in my left boob. Immediately my head goes into overdrive, imagining going back to treatment and trying to save my life. Of course I have no idea, but this is why I wrote this book to help others understand that the worry never goes away. It is there bubbling under the surface, ready to boil over with the slightest sign of anything out of the usual. I take a picture of Bea's rash and send it to the breast nurse. The nurse replies quickly and reassures me that she thinks it is just the area of the skin around my wound healing rather than a rash. After a few days monitoring the area, it subsides and I once again go back to low-level alert, but it really is exhausting being on this post-cancer roller coaster.

KINDLY BLUNT ADVICE

Being post-cancer does not mean you can just forget about the fight to become cancer free. It is normal to worry with every ache or pain and I like to think of it as my inner health-and-safety officer being a little over zealous. But that safety officer could well alert me to something I do need to take note of, so I need to pay attention.
If you are a friend or family member of someone post-cancer, please don't assume they will just bounce back to their former

self. Of course, anyone who has been fortunate enough to get the "no sign of cancer" is grateful, but with it comes a tonne of worry and anxiety. Being told "you should be happy now" will never help to make a cancer survivor worry any less.

DEM BONES

"I am determined cancer is not going to take the old me away"

Infusions

I was pushed fast through menopause during my chemotherapy, and although that was hard, I do appreciate that I was of an age when that would happen naturally, just a lot slower. I am grateful, however, that when my cancer was diagnosed, I didn't need to worry about fertility, as I already have children. It was a harsh way to go through menopause, but not as harsh as younger women who, through treatment, lose their fertility far too early in life. Now I am finished with my treatment, my oncology team recommends I don't take HRT to alleviate symptoms. Therefore, it is down to me to keep myself as healthy as possible. I know that menopause will have an effect on my bones, cardiovascular and brain function. I therefore decide to help myself age the best way I can. I have not yet convinced myself that I will reach sixty years of age, but I decide to put that to the back of my head just in case I do keep the shadow of cancer away! If I get to sixty, I need to be looking fabulous.

Bone strength declines as we get older and right now I have no idea what the state of my bones is. After many rounds of chemotherapy and fast-track menopause, my worry is I may have lost bone density. I am having zoledronic acid infusions every six months to keep my bones strong and to deter cancer from returning there, but I still have no idea what condition they have been left in. Back in 2018, before cancer was a word in my personal vocabulary, I was already interested in my bone density, so I went for a private scan up in London. Fortunately, the results were brilliant for my age. My bone strength was in the highest percentile for my age, and my muscle-to-fat ratio was high. My weight was well within normal limits and I felt great. I hate cancer for changing my body, but dwelling on that is not going to help get it sorted. Today I am off to London for another scan at the same clinic. I am going to find out my current bone density, but also how much my muscle-to-fat ratio has changed. Chemotherapy, steroids, menopause and lack of movement has meant I am two stone heavier than the last scan so I am dreading this. The scan does not take long to do and soon it is time to get the results. I will start by sharing with you the good news. My bones are strong and above average for my age. This is such good news after having chemotherapy. Next the not-so-good news: my muscle-to-fat ratio has changed drastically. I have far more fat than I should have.

I travel home with mixed emotions. Of course, I am happy that my bone density is good, but the huge change in my body shape is drastic and naturally I blame it all on cancer and all that comes with it. Feelings of it not being fair rise inside me and although I am not proud of those thoughts, they are real. Once I am over the shock I decide to focus on making changes. I am determined cancer is not going to take the old me away. I call the scan centre and book in another scan for eight months' time, then plan out a regime of weight training and healthy eating. To increase my muscle mass I have been advised to eat more protein and lift weights.

KINDLY BLUNT ADVICE

Bone strength is important and if I put my osteopathic hat on, I am able to tell you how important it is to think about your own bone density. Osteopenia and osteoporosis are terms for weakened bone structure, which predisposes you to fractures of all bones in your body, including your spine. Male or female, you will naturally lose bone density as you age and ideally you should build your bone density in your younger years. Most people reach their peak bone mass at around 25 to 30 years of age. Bone mass also has a link to your genetics. However, it is not too late to slow down loss of bone density. To help maintain your bone mass, do regular weight-bearing exercise, eat a healthy diet, don't smoke and reduce alcohol consumption. These are all things that will benefit your overall health too, not just your bones. Smile lots, as that always makes you feel good too.

Time To Start Living

FREEDOM

"I hardly think about cancer and I feel free"

Escape

I am about to escape from normal life for five whole weeks. Eddie and I are off in our campervan, for a five-week tour of eastern and northern England. We plan to visit beautiful coasts, historic towns and scenic countryside as we make our way up to Northumberland. I feel free, with no more hospital checks on the horizon. I can't wait to just be me, away with Eddie, living life. It's time to get in our campervan and leave the hospitals, consultants, and black shadow of cancer behind me. We set off, visiting multiple places along the coast. We have a vague idea of the direction we want to travel, but we only plan a few days in advance as we go. The freedom is liberating after being so controlled by my healthcare appointments. We travel to Colchester, Cromer, Epworth, Whitby, Beadnell Bay, Nunnykirk, Barnard Castle, Towcester, Stratford, Cirencester, Devizes, Wells and finally Wallingford where Eddie was born.

We purchased our campervan just before I was diagnosed with breast cancer. "Effy", as we call her, became my place of solace during the weeks of chemotherapy. I would have my chemotherapy on Fridays every week and the day after we would set off in the van, keeping close to home in case of an emergency. Very often we did not return until the following Tuesday, just before I was due back in hospital for bloods being taken before my next infusion. Despite the ravages of chemotherapy, the van was a place to escape. I didn't have to pretend to anyone that I was well. I could sleep when I wanted, eat what I wanted and the best bit was rising early to sit outside, wrapped up in an old sleeping bag, to watch the sunrise. I felt at peace in the van and I still do to this day. I get in it, immediately relax and the black shadow disappears.

As I want to do everything I can to stay healthy, I commit to doing alternate days of weights and yoga as well as getting daily steps or bike rides in whilst we are away. It is fabulous to do my exercise outside the van, although I do get some funny looks from other campers on occasions. If it rains I can roll out an exercise mat down the middle of the van as it is the perfect size. For a whole five weeks I hardly think about cancer and I feel free. It is like being in a protective bubble and I dread going home and the reality of that black shadow returning.

YEARLY CHECK

"Sixty minutes of my precious life is gone"

Poor Bea

We have arrived back from our five-week adventure touring England and immediately I am worrying about my health. I am conscious I have not received the invitation to my now yearly mammogram. I am sure it was due in March and it is now June. Poor Bea still has to endure this examination yearly, as the medical team tell me her risk of developing cancer is likely to be increased, so despite previously being my perfect boob she still needs close monitoring. As it happens, the hospital reports back that her mammogram is not due until August so I am too early, but they seem quite concerned that I have not had my yearly oncology check-up, informing me I should have had it two months ago. It should have been an automatic invitation, but it seems my name was not added to the list by the consultant. I think back to the disorganised consultant I saw last year and I am not totally surprised she missed allocating my repeat check. Within an hour, I have a face-to-face consultant appointment booked in a few days. Yes, another reality check that they are not prepared for me to leave things any longer than necessary.

Smoke Coming Out Of My Ears

Here I am again, back in the outpatients' waiting room that services multiple outpatient clinics. I have spent hours of my life waiting in this room. My appointments are very rarely on time and of course I am sympathetic to their busy schedules, but that does not stop me again pondering the irony of them saving my life then wasting precious minutes of it too.

I have been waiting 45 minutes and it makes me guess I am seeing the same consultant as last year. She was very late then too and you may remember me complaining earlier in this book. I have sat here now for over 45 minutes plus an extra 15 minutes because I didn't want to be late. If I had been late there are many signs up telling me my appointment will be cancelled. I am conscious I have kept up my side of the deal by being on time. An hour of my precious life is gone and not one person has told me there is a delay and explained how long I may have to wait. I am an expert in customer care with my previous ownership of a large multi-healthcare clinic that ran to time. It's simple customer care to tell the person so that they can manage their expectations if you are running late. However, nothing is said to me and as I watch every other person in that waiting room go in and then leave after appointments. I am getting more and more angry. Finally, with just me left in the waiting room, as I watch the nurse put her coat on and go to leave for the day, I ask if I have been forgotten. This nurse is not involved with my clinic timing, but dutifully she goes off to check once I tell her it is now an hour since my appointment time with no communication. I think she can see the smoke coming out of my ears.

After some inaudible chat the nurse comes back and tells me I will be seen in 10 minutes. The steam in my head subsides, but honestly this could have been dealt with better. Finally, I get in to see the consultant and it is the same person as my previous visit; once again, I just can't get over her disorganisation. I ponder that I could have spent the last wasted hour of my life putting some order into her clinic room. At least I could have written down my name, as she is not immediately sure who I am, as I sit waiting for her to scroll on her PC. Despite the drag on my time and the worryingly disorganised approach, this doctor does have excellent examination skills and she finally reports everything seems normal. I don't own up that I used to be an examiner for osteopathic students so I recognise good palpation. Perhaps I should have given her a mark out of 10.

Despite being checked by the consultant, as I walk back to my car I worry that my yearly check is only a manual examination of my chest area rather than a scan of my whole body. How would they know that cancer isn't raging through my body unchecked with just this method? I know how small a rogue cell is and how fast it could spread without my knowledge and it does make me uneasy. Despite a positive manual check, that dark shadow is behind me and I worry more than ever that it will reappear when I least expect it. However, I come away from the appointment with some relief and also the idea that the consultant desperately needs a personal assistant to organise her. She is obviously highly intelligent in medical matters to be a consultant, but her admin and time-keeping skills are lacking. I take a reality check and realise I prefer it this way around than the other. I can put up with disorganised when her medical skills are hopefully keeping me safe.

LOU'S HEN

"I really do appreciate the little things"

Hens And Cakes

Today is all about my daughter and her second hen celebration, for those that didn't attend her previous hen weekend away. I am on duty to provide an afternoon tea and I am in my element. I love baking and any chance I get I will make the family a cake or pudding. Baking has always been a type of therapy for me and a distraction from everything else going on in my world. I think back to the times during my chemotherapy when I could hardly stand at the kitchen work surface and when baking resulted in hot flushes and needing a chair to sit on every five minutes. During chemotherapy I missed being well enough to bake, but this weekend I have energy and lots of it. I rush about making everything perfect and it's a joy to do so. I really do appreciate the little things these days.

What I haven't mentioned is the elephant in the room. This morning I got an NHS letter through the door. I know it is the results from my yearly mammogram on Bea a few weeks ago and I am terrified. This may not be logical terror as it is Bea who was scanned, who didn't have cancer, and I have no other symptoms to make me suspicious, but I still remember the day back in 2021 when my routine mammogram results dropped on the mat. Without a care in the world I opened the letter, never expecting to be called back and never once thinking I would have cancer. I decide, very quickly, that I am not going to open that letter right now. I have a day of fun ahead of me with my daughter and her hen party. I am not about to open this letter with a chance that it may contain bad news. I stash the letter away without sharing with anyone it has arrived. One extra day is not going to make a difference, if it has come back positive for cancer. I am not going to ruin my daughter's day.

The hen goes well. On the most glorious summer afternoon we spend the day drinking too much fizz and eating cake. A perfect day. Just like the cancer shadow, the letter is at the back of my mind. Even when the guests have gone, I can't make myself open it. It has been the most beautiful day and I am not about to spoil it. Finally, a whole 48 hours after getting the letter, I share with Eddie that I have hidden it away. I ask him to sit with me as I open it. I don't have cancer, or at least Bea doesn't. She really is the best boob a girl could ask for. I have no real assurance that cancer is not travelling elsewhere in my body, but it does seem like I can relax again for a while. What a fabulous weekend this was.

KINDLY BLUNT ADVICE

Remember to appreciate the little things in your life. It can be easy to take the simple things in life for granted. Take 10 minutes to be grateful for all that you have, and if you want a real boost, bake a cake for yourself and friends. Don't forget to cut yourself a large slice.

BARBIE BODY

"Renaming my boobs Pinky and Perky"

Embrace Every Wrinkle

Who would have thought that I would be sitting here telling you I am off to see my plastic surgeon today? I feel like those wealthy people that have money to get "things done". They have their own personal surgeon who does nips and tucks to try to prevent ageing. Personally I am not sure it works, but if it makes them happy then who am I to tell them to embrace every wrinkle as a privilege? Actually, forget that, of course I would loudly tell them to embrace every wrinkle as a privilege.

My surgery could be seen as vanity, but in my mind I have replaced what was taken. Agnes was surgically removed and that left me lopsided. I was also too lazy to be mucking about with a fake boob and worrying about how clothes would fit. It does affect you psychologically when your body is chopped about, and I hope it makes me feel less like a cancer victim and more like me again.

Here I sit with a "boob job" and "tummy tuck". I never would have considered any sort of plastic surgery prior to the ravages of cancer and treatment, but here I am off to see my plastic surgeon for some tweaks to the work already done. My surgeon's work has been amazing. Removing the fat I had from my stomach to create a new boob where Agnes once sat is incredible and the results are way beyond my expectations. It actually looks like a boob rather than a lump of my belly stuck on my chest, which is how I thought it might look. Moving forward, it is likely I will also have a nipple tattoo on the new boob.

Today I am off for belly boob, Agnes's replacement, resizing. Eddie will come with me today and as always I am grateful. Any trip back to a hospital is always a trigger for me and in my experience no appointment goes quite as I thought it would. It is seven months since my reconstruction surgery and now the surgical team want to take a look and, if necessary, discuss levelling things up. I am just happy I have another boob bump where Agnes was, but today they are going to make sure Bea and my new belly boob match. It takes months for things to settle and today they are going to see if I need liposuction to make Bea slightly smaller. I am not sure how she will react to that, as I know she is very happy with her bonus lift during surgery. Plastic surgery, a tattoo and liposuction I am starting to feel like an A-lister trying to keep my looks. Prior to being diagnosed with cancer, I was very happy to grow old gracefully without surgical help and always believed every wrinkle is an honour to be celebrated. I had a mum's belly with many stretch marks that were my proudly earned badge of Mum honour but here I am today with a rebuilt body. I will admit I look a bit like a patchwork quilt and I am proud some of those Mum stretch marks are now moved to my chest. In the great scheme of things, I am aware just how lucky I am and how I will be forever grateful for everyone that has been part of my survival and recovery journey. Modern medicine really is amazing.

My Precious Life

Here I am again waiting for my appointment, losing a few more minutes of my precious life. Of course, I am forever grateful but today the overrun wait time is ninety minutes. This time however, unlike my last consultant visit, the nurses are quick to inform me that my clinic is running late, it seems all the consultants on this floor are overrunning, as the waiting room is packed. It is hot outside and one little fan is not making much difference to a group of disgruntled patients. The TV screen that usually shows daily programmes has a blank screen, so there is not even any entertainment while we wait. Thankfully, I get told we can go away and come back an hour after my original appointment time, so we quickly slope off for a coffee. As luck would have it, this week is the start of the Olympics in Paris and as we walk through an empty waiting room downstairs, we see the TV is on showing the day's events. We grab a drink and head back to the cooler, empty area and watch the Olympics. This is good customer care as I have been fully informed and I have the choice to fill in the time in a less wasteful way. Finally, the nurse comes down to find me. The consultant is ready. My usual plastic surgeon is on holiday, so I am to see an associate. I am not sure how this is going to go. How will she know what to do?

Since this all started, I have had photos taken of my body, namely my chest and abdomen area. In my book *Agnes, Bea, Cancer and Me*, I share my photoshoot in the depths of the hospital. A boob model I am not, but I sure rock a photoshoot with my battered body. I have had a photoshoot done at this hospital a couple of times now, once before my reconstruction surgery and once after. Today's consultant has my pictures on her screen. Not a pretty sight, but of course she is used to viewing pictures like that. I get asked about my health and they seem really pleased when I tell them I feel great, I am back training and I have no problems. Without saying as much, it seems they wished this for the previous patient. "Shame you couldn't share your story with the last lady," was said. I am very aware I have got through this reconstruction well and the outcome is fantastic. Today gratitude is rising up instead of the dark shadow.

I am ready to stop having my body feel like an object, but of course in this check-up there has to be a point when I am asked to undress to show my reconstruction areas. The medical staff are kind, caring and consider my modesty at every move, but it does make me feel like my body now belongs to the medical team. I have perfected a method of shutting off my mind to the process whilst the discussions and scrutiny of my body are going on. It is now three years since I was pulled back in after an abnormal routine mammogram. For the last three years I have been "flashing" at medical staff, I have been on at least four boob photoshoots in two different hospitals and multiple surgeons have worked on my chest area either removing cancerous tissue or adding belly fat back to the area. Prior to this, I was never a person to expose my body. It seems I am now a changed person. Just call me "Flasher Bullen".

Today the consultant takes a look at Bea and belly boob and she is impressed. I can see by her face and her comments that she is pleased with the change that has taken place since my last visit six months ago. I now have two shapely boobs. She comments that the new one is slightly fuller and then seems to struggle to verbally express how it compares with Bea. Bea was given an uplift, but still is not quite as perky as belly boob. A shame really as I was thinking of renaming my boobs Pinky and Perky. I help the consultant find her words by announcing that "Bea is sagging a little." She looks relieved and nods as I fill in the blanks for her. I don't care, as far as I am concerned, they both look great and inside I smile at her slight discomfort in describing the scenario.

I am delighted to report that I don't need any more plastic surgery. After discussion with the consultant, we agree that the outcome of my reconstruction surgery is good and I am feeling very fortunate. Not everyone gets the results they want on the first attempt. All I need to do now is to get a nipple tattoo put onto belly boob and

I am ready to go. I have never wanted a tattoo as they are just not my thing. I admire them on others but not for me. How I have changed. A boob job, a tummy tuck and now a tattoo! Who is this new person? This had better make me cool. I very much doubt that I am in any way cool, but I do think I may be on my way to a Barbie body. Excuse me while I double over laughing.

Eddie seems relieved as we leave the clinic room. He doesn't often comment on my choices, but he admits he is glad I am not going to have more surgery. He is, after all, the person that looks after me when I come out of hospital. He has seen me struggle in the weeks after the operations and I am glad he does not have to go through that again. I am relieved that I can continue getting stronger and fitter without further surgery and the long recovery that comes with it. We jump in the car and start to drive home. After about 15 minutes my tears flow. The realisation that I am getting to the end of all this shit finally hits me like a sledgehammer. No more operations and only one more zoledronic acid infusion in January. After that, I will just have to come back for yearly in-person checks and mammograms for the next few years. Finally, I can see the light at the end of this long and shitty tunnel and all I have to do is stay cancer free. I have no control over the cancer, but what I can do is keep living life to the full and stay positive. I didn't realise what a big day today was, but the relief is huge. I want to get off this rollercoaster and forget this all happened, and the less time I have to be in hospital being checked, the slower the rollercoaster gets and soon, I hope, I can get off and never go back.

Tattoo

It's a few days since my check-up and something has been bugging me. The tattoo. It just doesn't sit right with me to get a nipple tattoo on my belly boob. I have had enough of hospital visits and, to be honest, I don't need it. Belly boob will always be just that, a belly boob, and even with a tattoo I will never consider it a real replacement for Agnes. What I have is good enough, a boob shape, which I don't need to mimic a real boob. Although most tattoos are safe, I just don't want to chance infection or not liking the result. I am happy and I have decided it is time to stop any more treatment. I have just emailed the hospital and cancelled the appointment. I am hopeful I never have to return to this specialised plastic surgery hospital, despite all their amazing and life-changing work. Now I need to get on with my life. I don't want any more work done on my body. Instead I want to walk away, head held high, with thanks for all they have done.

MOTHER OF THE BRIDE

"A day I didn't cause anyone any worry"

Exactly Three Years

It is August 2024 and today my daughter gets married. I am so excited, I just can't write enough words to explain how good it feels to get to this occasion and be well. It is exactly three years since I started my first round of chemotherapy. This time three years ago, nobody could give me a guarantee I would survive; instead, I was put on weekly chemotherapy and for six months I held my breath, hoping I could turn things around. If the cancer had not been found early enough at a routine mammogram, I am in little doubt that I would not be here today. Even though I am not religious, I feel blessed to be alive and able to go to my daughter's wedding. I am also acutely aware not everyone with a diagnosis like mine is so fortunate.

When I was first diagnosed, I thought it was the end. I cried as the nurse explained there were no guarantees, but that starting chemotherapy and a mastectomy was my best chance of survival. I was frantic with worry that I would miss key moments in my children's lives. I thought about writing letters for key moments in their lives to know I was with them even if they could not see me. I had nightmares of my chair at both my children's weddings being empty and me being a cause of sadness on days they should be celebrating. However, today I will be sitting in the Mother of the Bride seat. I am almost back to my normal size, my hair is now fully returned and I have a hairstyle I chose rather than just trying to grow it back. My nails are painted, my dress is hanging ready and my shoes are of course fabulous! I feel well, I feel strong and I know I am going to enjoy my day. Luckily before my makeup is done I shed a few happy tears as I get ready. I am so fortunate and today is going to be one of the best days of my life, I just know it.

The Wedding

I get to enjoy a full day with my daughter and it begins by arriving at her house early to get ready with her and the bridesmaids. It's a fun morning with just the four of us and the beautician making us all look fabulous, glasses of fizz and plenty of laughs. The sun is shining and it is all perfect. I am so grateful I survived to see this happen. Somehow it gives me some peace for whatever is around the corner for my health. A milestone reached and a day I didn't cause anyone any worry. The time soon comes for us all to leave and travel to the venue. We arrive and it's all perfect. The weather is so good that the ceremony can be outside. I make my way to my seat to watch the celebrations unfold with so much gratitude I feel I may explode. Yes, of course, I did make sure my beautiful shoes were on show in the aisle before the bride arrived.

It is a perfect day of family, friends, fun and smiles. We dance our way into the early hours and I feel this is the perfect place to end this book. I am so happy, my family are happy and life just feels perfect. I still have a shadow behind me, but in front of me I feel a shining light of life that I shall be living to the full as long as the universe allows. I am so grateful for my story having a happy ending and my heart is heavy for all those who are not so fortunate.

In their honour I will keep living the best life I can with gratitude and a smile every day.

KINDLY BLUNT GRATITUDE

Thank you for taking the time to read my story. Writing this has proved to be its own form of therapy for me and I hope, if you are going through a similar journey or know someone who is, that it has given you hope. This is a message for us all – please live life to the full, smile every day, keep the shadows behind you and face the sun as you go. Helen x

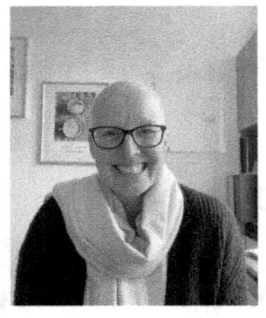
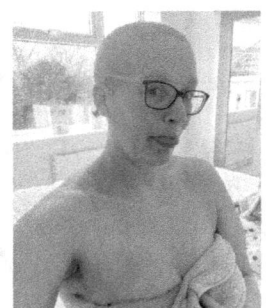
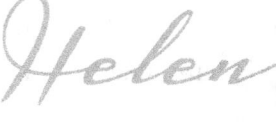
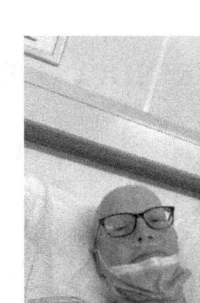
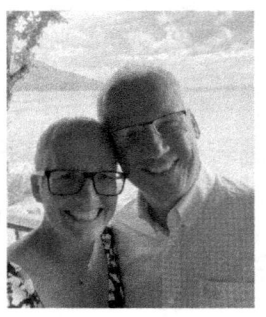
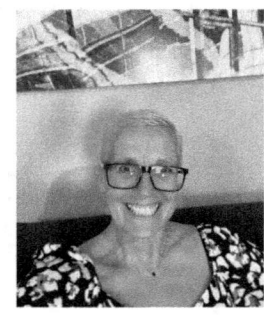
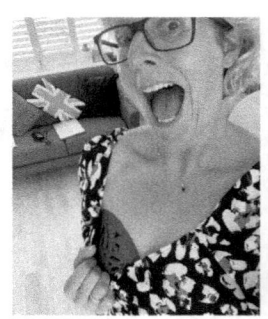
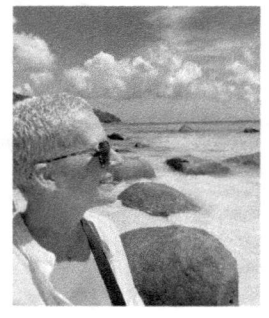
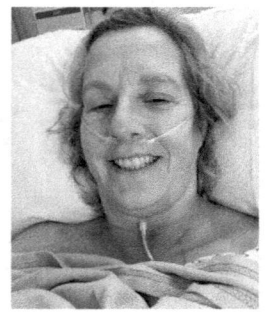
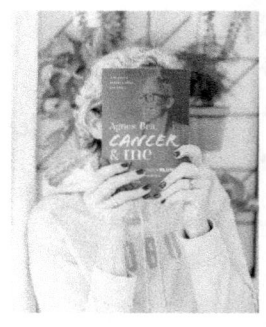

KIN♡LY BLUNT

Helen

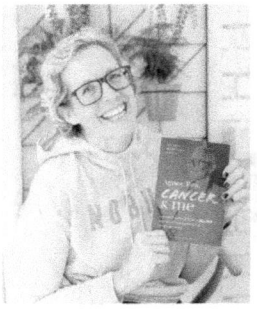
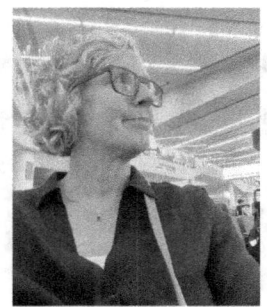
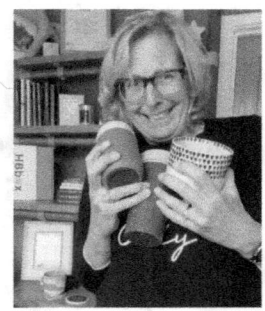
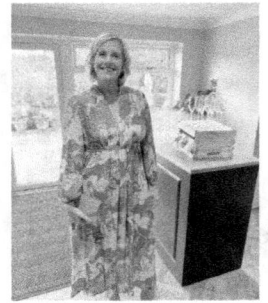
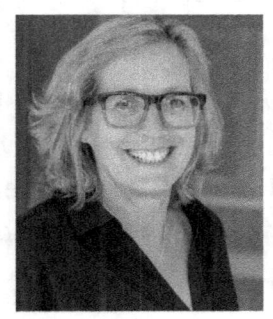
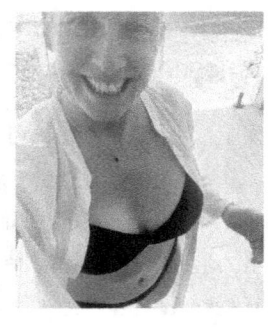
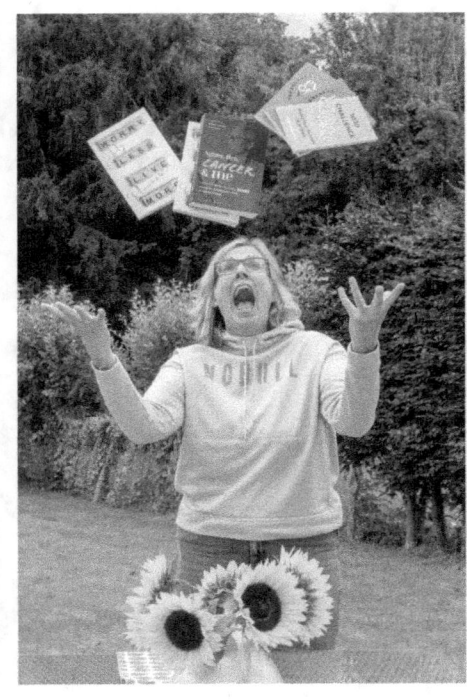
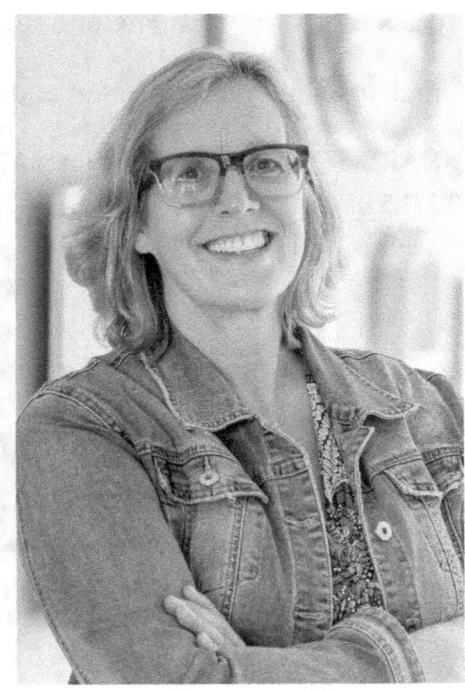

LEAVE A REVIEW

Thank you for reading my book, Me, Bea, Cancer Free, I hope you enjoyed it and found it helpful too.

This book was written to help others, and I would like to make sure many people get to read it. If you enjoyed the book, I would be really grateful if you would take the time to leave a review on Amazon. The more reviews the book gets, the more visible it will become on the Amazon platform.

Once you have left your review, ping me an email so I can say thank you personally: **helen@helenbullen.com**

Much love and thanks, Helen and Bea x

SHARE YOUR REVIEW ON AMAZON AND OTHER ONLINE RETAILERS

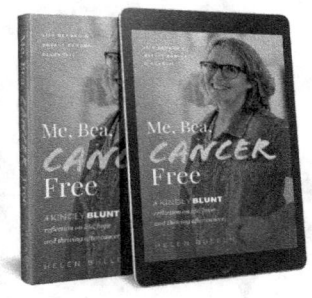

GRATITUDE

A NOTE OF THANKS

Just like in *Agnes, Bea, Cancer and Me*, there are so many people to thank – and honestly, words will never feel quite enough. I'm incredibly grateful for the amazing people I have in my life, especially those who went above and beyond when things got tough (and let's be honest, they got *really* tough). You know who you are and please know this: I will never forget your kindness, your encouragement, or your strength when mine was running low.

Many of my superheroes have already heard me say thank you in person, probably more than once but I want to say it again here, in black and white, because your support helped me not just get through this chapter of my life, but also helped me bring this book into the world.

Thank you for walking with me. For cheering me on. For believing in me when I needed it most. I am forever grateful.

MEDICAL TEAM

There are far too many individuals to personally mention that have helped me go through reconstruction and recover on the other side. Each one has a special place in my heart for the knowledge they have taken time to study to enable people like me to benefit from their amazing work. From specialised surgeons to trolley porters they have all taken care of me and I am truly so grateful. These are the staff that have helped rebuild my body and keep a check on whether the cancer has returned. I have to thank them all.

ADVANCED READER TEAM

Huge thanks must be given to all the people who volunteered to read the book early and give their valued feedback. You are all awesome. Thank you for giving up your time to help make sure this book was published at its very best.

DESIGN/EDITING TEAM

It takes many people to produce a book that is worthy to sit on your shelf and I am thankful for everyone on this list. (Even me for learning a new skill and implementing it in this books design)

Editing: Melanie Scott – https://reedsy.com/melanie-scott

Proof Reading: Eddie Sinden (AKA my husband, who has a hidden skill I am now utilising)

Book Design: Helen Bullen Publishing - https://helenbullen.com/

Cover and Interior design (original idea): Becky's GraphicDesign , LLC – https://beckysgraphicdesign.com

Cover Photo: Andy Newbold – https://www.newboldphotography.com/

Eddie Judd: https://eddiejuddphotography.co

HB Branding and Logos: Jessica Lynn – https://www.jessicalynndesign.com/

Thank you.

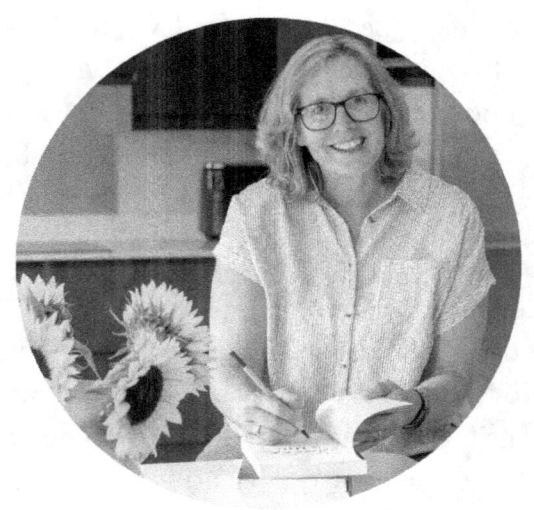

ABOUT THE AUTHOR

Helen Bullen is many things: a straight talking business mentor, a retired award winning osteopath, a best selling author, and most recently, a breast cancer survivor with a stubborn streak and a sense of humour that not even chemo could crush.

With over 20 years of experience running her own successful businesses in both bricks-and-mortar clinics and online, Helen knows a thing or two about building something from the ground up. She is the founder of HBClub, HBInspired and the HBRetreat, where she helps business owners cut through the noise, get real about their goals and take action. No fluff, no faffing, no excuses. Her philosophy is simple: you can achieve anything when you commit to it. And yes, she means anything.

In 2021, life threw Helen one of its biggest curveballs when she was diagnosed with stage 3 Triple Negative breast cancer. What followed was months of treatment, multiple surgeries and a fierce determination to not just survive but thrive. She wrote her first cancer memoir, *Agnes, Bea, Cancer and Me*, to share the raw, real and occasionally ridiculous realities of life with cancer. Now, in her follow up book "*Me, Bea, Cancer Free*", she explores life after treatment, the unexpected challenges of getting back to normal and what it really means to move forward when nothing feels the same.

These days Helen lives her version of the good life. She works the hours she chooses, mentors the people she genuinely loves to help and says yes to what brings her joy and no to everything else. Her story is one of grit, grace and a whole lot of humour, and she shares it to support others who are navigating their own after cancer journey.

You can find her books on Amazon and in all good bookshops. You will also find her, coffee in hand, cheering others on because if she has learned anything, it is that life is too short not to go after what matters most.

Helen

JOIN MY COMMUNITY

Would you like to hear more from me? I love to write and not just books. I also like to connect with readers.

Happy Business Builders

Join my weekly email list for small business owners. Each week I share business tips, ideas, motivation with a sprinkle of fun direct to your inbox.
Just ask to join using this link https://helenbullen.kartra.com/page/HappyBusinessBuilder

Substack

Join me on a platform where I will write about anything that takes my fancy, from extracts from any new books I am writing to my views on everyday things. As always, I will be Kindly Blunt and try to add fun to it along the way.

https://helenbullenauthor.substack.com/publish/home

Email Me

If you want to get in touch with me personally, then please contact me via email helen@helenbullen.com

Social Media

Another great way to get in touch is to find me on my social media platforms. See below:

FACEBOOK https://www.facebook.com/helenbullenuk

INSTAGRAM https://www.instagram.com/helenbullenuk/

TIKTOK https://www.tiktok.com/@helenbullenuk

LINKEDIN https://www.linkedin.com/in/helenbullen

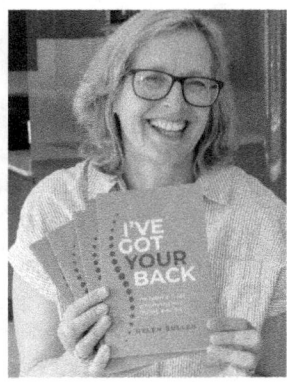
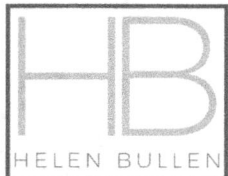
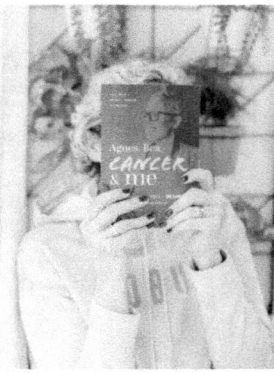
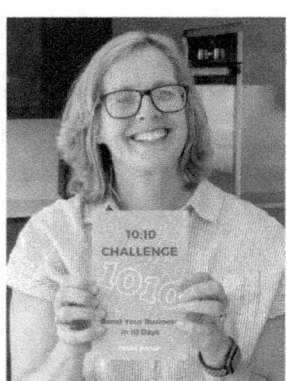
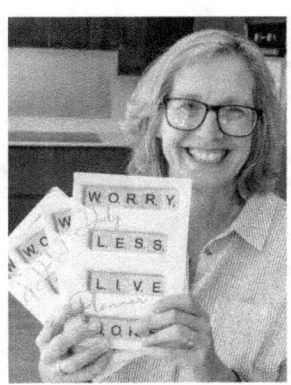
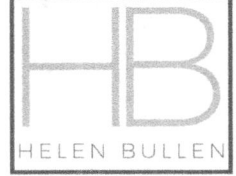
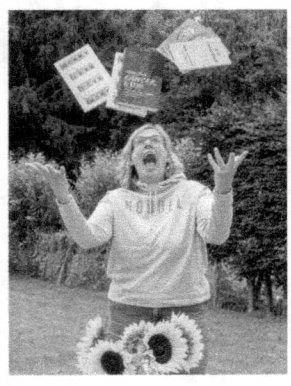
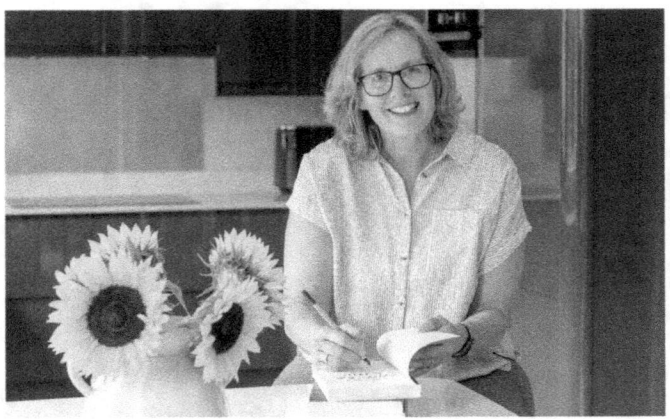

Check out all my books on Amazon and all good book stores.

A KINDLY BLUNT
BOOK

www.ingramcontent.com/pod-product-compliance
Lightning Source LLC
Chambersburg PA
CBHW071244070526
44583CB00017B/2313